MW00781050

Week 26

A Memoir of Hope, Faith,
and Perseverance

JENNIFER ALVES BERNARDO

Paperback: 979-8-9901569-0-6
Hardcover: 979-8-9901569-1-3
Ebook: 979-8-9901569-2-0

www.week26.com

Contents

this book is dedicated to
my three children and to the millions
of families around the world with babies
in the neonatal intensive care unit.

Out of respect for their privacy, I used very few people's names in this book, but there are many who played an integral part in helping our family get through such a difficult yet triumphant time.

CHAPTER 1

This Can't Be Happening

I awoke with my heart pounding. A faint glow from the hallway crept under my bedroom door. Sitting up in bed, I looked over at my husband Joe, lost in a deep sleep. Still entangled in my dreams, I couldn't quite get my bearings, but I knew something wasn't right. There was a shift—in my body, in the air around me. I couldn't name it, but I could feel it.

Angelina, our five-year-old daughter, was sleeping in the room next door. The digital clock on my bedside table read 2:02 a.m. Everyone in the house was quiet and at peace. Everyone but me.

This wasn't the first time this had happened. In fact, for the past few months, nightmares had plagued me. I could never remember exactly what they were about, but I always woke up terrified, in a cold sweat, with my pulse racing the way it was now. My doctor had said this pattern was normal during pregnancy, as my body's heightened levels of progesterone could result in vivid dreams, but I wished it would stop—until I realized that my current reality was even more horrifying.

At first, I felt as if someone had tossed a bucket of warm water on me. My nightgown, my underwear, my bed—everything was soaked. But then, as my foggy brain cleared, I knew I was bleeding before I even turned on the light.

Earlier that week, light spotting had sent me to my high-risk obstetrician for a checkup. I was 26 weeks pregnant with twins. The doctors told me that I had developed placenta previa, meaning that my placenta was partially blocking my birth canal. But because it was a mild case, the problem would likely resolve on its own. As a woman's uterus expands during pregnancy, a low placenta often shifts upward to the top of the uterus, leaving the cervix clear for childbirth. Spotting was okay, my doctor had said. But she had advised me that if I ever experienced a rush of blood down my legs, I should go to the hospital immediately.

Jumping out of bed now, I charged into my bathroom and flipped on the light, forcing myself to look down. My inner thighs were bright red, and I had left bloody footprints on the tile floor. My eyes followed the tracks back to my bed and the dark stain that had spread across my sheets. For the time being, the bleeding seemed to have subsided, but I knew it could start again anytime. So, I hastily rinsed my legs and feet in the bathtub, rushed back to Joe's side, and shook his shoulder.

"Babe, wake up! We need to go to the hospital—now!"

"What's the matter?" Joe mumbled.

I sobbed as I spoke to him. "I'm bleeding—a lot. I think it's stopped for now, but something is really wrong. We need to go!"

Without another word, Joe pulled on clothes and called our neighbor to ask her to come over while we went to the hospital. Trying to stay calm so as to not worry them, I called my parents and, while downplaying the situation, asked them to take over from our neighbor as quickly as they could. In the meantime, I cleaned myself up more thoroughly, put a pad in my underwear, got dressed, and went down the hall to Angelina's room.

She looks so warm and safe, I thought, a lump forming in my throat as I stood beside her bed watching her sleep. I hoped her excitement about finding my parents at our house the next morning would outweigh any fear she had about the fact that her parents had disappeared in the middle of the night. I trusted that my mother would tell her I had gone to the doctor and would be home soon.

As I ran my fingers through Angelina's long, silky brown hair, brushing a strand off her forehead, I thought, *I will do anything to make sure my twins are safe and peaceful, just like their sister is at this very moment.* "I love you so much," I whispered, leaning down to kiss my daughter's forehead. But I couldn't stay any longer for fear that my bleeding would restart, so I hurried outside, where Joe was waiting for me in the car.

While we drove, I barely noticed the abandoned streets, slick with January frost. All I could think about were my babies and whether they were alive and well. At my last visit, they were each not even a foot long.

Hands shaking, I dialed my OB. Unfortunately, she was not assigned to the nearest hospital, where we were headed, but she assured me, "You're doing the right thing. You'll be in good hands there. Don't worry—I really don't think you're going to have these babies today. Just call me if you need anything."

It all sounded good, but was she just feeding me false hope because she knew how apprehensive I was? Ever since I had found out that I was pregnant with twins, I had been battling unrelenting anxiety. Unlike my first pregnancy with Angelina, this one had me on edge for some reason, as if something bad was going to happen at any moment. Everyone knows that in a birth with multiples, you have a higher risk of complications. I kept having the same train of thought: *I can't believe that I have two babies inside me. I'm so petite—how are they going to fit inside my stomach as they grow? Am I going to have to have a C-section? I've never even experienced surgery. What if they come early?*

I typically assume even difficult situations will work out eventually, and so far, I had no medical evidence that any of these what-if scenarios would come to fruition. All of the genetic tests we had done had come back normal, the twins' growth was right on track, and my body seemed to be doing a fine job of nurturing them. Still, my usual optimism and rational mind just weren't strong enough to overpower my unease.

I was often hesitant to verbalize my fears to Joe, especially when I knew he was trying to get his own head around the twins' impending birth, but he always defaulted to a position of strength and stoicism if anyone in his family was in danger or distress. Now, keeping his left hand on the steering wheel, he reached over with his right and clasped my hand.

I tried to focus on soaking up his support, but as we neared the hospital, I couldn't stop my frenetic thoughts: *My babies have to be all right. It's way too early for them to be born. I have to think positively. I have to keep it together and hope for the best.* I cradled my belly in my hands, eagerly anticipating the twins' tiny kicks. But I felt nothing. No movement. Only the terror gnawing at my insides.

CHAPTER 2

Putting Away the Past

―――――

With four months left until your babies arrive, you're supposed to be preparing the nursery, picking names, buying baby
clothes, and planning for the future—not speeding down the
interstate in the middle of the night because your pregnant
wife is bleeding in the seat next to you.

When Jenny woke me, a switch flipped in my mind. My
emotions and fear turned off, and a vigorous strength turned
on. This happened anytime my family needed me—the more
serious the challenge, the stronger I was.

I've been this way since I was a child. As a one-year-old,
I immigrated to the United States with my parents, who both
came from small villages in Portugal. Married at 19 and 24,
respectively, my mother and father saw each other 10 times or

less at the doorstep of my grandfather's house before they were wed. My mother probably did it to get out of her village; my dad was just coming out of the army and figured it was time to settle down and find a wife. In my mother, he found a beautiful woman with big dreams of moving to America.

Once they immigrated, however, any grandiose visions of a better life that my parents had entertained in Portugal quickly dissolved due to the many challenges they faced. Neither of them spoke English, and my father worked a demanding construction job six days a week to provide for his family, which expanded when my sister was born when I was five. To supplement my dad's income, my mother, who had envisioned a more sophisticated existence for herself, had to clean houses. Living in a different country, not speaking the language, and leaving her family behind, my mother oftentimes found herself struggling emotionally. I had an unstable childhood and didn't have an idyllic upbringing of riding bikes and playing catch in the backyard with my father; instead, I was frequently finding ways to let out my emotions. When I was really young, I couldn't understand why my dad was always working so much, so it was easy for me to be mad at him most of the time when, looking back, he was just a very hardworking man trying to provide for our family. As a child, I always found myself playing referee at home during arguments between my parents, when really I should have been playing outside and just being a kid. Things weren't much better for me at school, either. I got teased a lot because of things like my weight, my cultural differences, and the fact that no one could pronounce my name correctly, so I had to stand up for myself, which resulted in a lot of altercations. The unexpected benefit of these early hardships was that, whether I was wriggling out of holds during wrestling matches or withstanding the bullying I received at school for being "different," I developed grit and willpower that have only continued to grow in my adulthood. "Joe the Bull," people called me. After all, I am a Taurus. And my tenacity only intensified when I was fighting for someone I loved.

Although parts of my past were tough, I found ways around my stress like video games, playing soccer, martial arts, spending endless nights out with friends, or vacationing in Miami. Sundays were spent with extended family around the table, eating delicious meals that my mom had cooked. I also built countless memories traveling to Portugal during the summer months to spend time with my wider family. I was often found mountain biking with my cousins or hanging out at a café on the beach or in a small village. I loved nothing more than the smell of fresh bread in the mornings or waking up to the sounds of a rooster crowing at the break of dawn. Portugal was my escape—my home away from home. It brought me a sense of peace and tranquility, unlike my everyday life in America.

I was raised and culturally conditioned to believe that my duty as a Portuguese male was to make family a priority; protecting those you love went without saying. Today, nothing comes before being there for my family. It took me a long time and a lot of therapy to get to where I am today, and my primary goal now is to make sure that my wife and children don't have trauma in their own lives that will affect them later. So, while I may be sensitive and emotional by nature, the minute I'm under pressure, a switch flips in me and I'm able to turn off any anxiety, fears, and doubts I've ever had. The world can be falling apart around me, but I've got to be the rock, because if anyone sees me freaking out, everyone else is going to freak out too. It's as if suddenly I don't want anybody else to stand in front of me; I want everyone I love behind me so I can protect them.

And that's exactly what happened the night Jenny woke me to tell me she was bleeding. As soon as I got out of bed, I was focused entirely on keeping her calm, getting her into the car, and sharing any encouraging words I could. "Just try to relax," I said as I drove, not so fast as to alarm her, but fast enough to get her the care she needed as soon as possible. "We're around the best hospitals; we have the best medical care. Whatever's going on with you is probably nothing."

As soon as I got onto the highway, I made an executive decision not to spend the extra 20 minutes driving to the hospital where Jenny was supposed to deliver the twins. I knew all the hospital facilities in our region of Virginia and the hospital closest to our house had one of the best neonatal intensive care units (NICUs) in the area. Even though I was telling Jenny everything was fine, I said to myself, *If something goes wrong with these babies, this is the hospital I want to be at.*

I'm not proud of the way I reacted when I found out Jenny and I were having twins. I realize now that my response was partly attributable to shock and fear, and partly the result of my own mental health struggles at the time, which my parents' recent, bitter divorce had ignited. Now, as I drove to the hospital, I couldn't help but wonder whether I was to blame for what was happening to Jenny—as if karma was coming back to bite me in the ass for, at times, being so negative. While she sat quietly next to me in the car, most likely praying that our babies would be okay, I kept up my running monologue about how we were almost there and how we would all be fine. But all the while, I just kept thinking, *Lord, forgive me for my fears, but you can't do this to Jenny. She doesn't deserve this, and my babies don't deserve this either.*

At the hospital entrance, I put the car in park, smiled at Jenny, kissed her cheek, and darted to the front entrance to get her a wheelchair. As I rolled it back to the car, I thought, *Nothing in the past matters anymore. What matters is that my wife and children are okay, and I am going to do anything and everything I can to make that happen.*

CHAPTER 3

More Than We Bargained For

At 2:30 a.m., the women's center looked empty. Joe parked right out front and grabbed a wheelchair from inside the entrance. He pushed it over to the car, helped me into it, and then rolled me to the check-in desk. As soon as the receptionist emerged from a back room, he explained that I was 26 weeks pregnant with twins and had just bled profusely. "We need help right away," he said, and the woman quickly wheeled me through double doors into the nearest room in the triage area.

While Joe left to park the car in the hospital garage, a team of doctors and nurses swarmed me. Deft, expert hands began swabbing my arm, preparing it for an IV. My veins popped beneath the elastic tourniquet that they snapped onto my bicep.

As the nurse taped down my IV, she said, "Tell me what's going on."

I repeated what Joe had said at triage, adding that I had just been diagnosed with placenta previa. I had gone to my high-risk OB for a vaginal ultrasound three days earlier, on Tuesday, because I had started spotting. At that appointment, the doctor had confirmed that I had mild placenta previa. Typically, once placenta previa has been established, vaginal ultrasounds are not performed because the probe can prompt bleeding. In my case, however, when I returned to my doctor's office on Friday, the ultrasound tech inserted another probe into my birth canal. Now, I couldn't help but wonder whether those two ultrasounds were what had started my dramatic hemorrhage and landed me in the hospital.

As I explained to the nurse what had happened, she frowned. "They put a probe in you *after* they diagnosed you with previa?"

"Yes," I said.

"They should *not* have done that," she said. "It's too risky."

Really? I thought, bracing myself to bleed again at any second.

The nurse patted my arm. "Regardless, try not to worry too much. We'll take the best care of you and your babies that we possibly can. Your vitals are good, and I gave you some magnesium sulfate to help you avoid preterm labor. Now, let's check on these twins."

She smeared cold gel on my belly and wrapped a thick ultrasound band, equipped with two Doppler transducer probes to detect a heartbeat, around it.

"Do you think they're okay?" I asked. *Please, please let them be okay*, I added silently, my own heart pounding.

"That's what we're about to find out."

The nurse moved the probe slowly around my belly, searching for signs of life. At first, I heard only static and soft gurgles, but my eyes widened when I detected a faint thumping sound.

"There's the first heartbeat!" the nurse said, beaming at me.

As she secured the Doppler probe in place and started searching again, I thought, *One baby is alive. One. But what about my other baby? They both have to be okay. They just have to be. They're a package deal.* The only way everything would be okay would be if I heard the steady thudding of two little hearts inside me.

When Joe and I were trying to conceive another child, we expected only a single birth—the most statistically likely outcome. The discovery that we were having twins naturally triggered a flood of worries but also a flood of excitement, shock, and surprise. Waiting for the nurse to locate the other heartbeat, I could not imagine what our lives would be like now if something happened to one or the other.

Another weak "thump-thump" startled me out of my reverie.

"Looks like they're both doing great," the nurse said.

I exhaled in a rush. I hadn't even realized I was holding my breath. "But still… something happened," I said. "Why did I start bleeding? Will it happen again?" I had so many questions.

Rather than answering me, the nurse put her hand on my shoulder and said, "Hang tight." I focused on the light pressure of her fingers anchoring me in place. "We need to get you upstairs to run some more tests. But your babies are okay. Hold on to that."

Keeping the fetal heart monitor strapped to my abdomen, she wheeled my hospital bed out of the triage area and up to a spacious room on the second floor. Joe followed, holding my belongings. The streetlamps outside the window cast a yellow glow on us while we rehashed the past hour and listened to our babies' hearts beating steadily in the background. As the night dragged toward morning, Joe fell asleep on the couch. I tried to rest too, but I was afraid something would happen to me or the twins if I dozed off.

Just before sunrise, I felt it again: streams of blood pouring down my legs, as if a faucet had been turned on full blast. I woke Joe as I pressed the call button over and over.

A nurse dashed to my bedside, gave me more medicine, and began cleaning me up. Strangely, I wasn't in any physical pain; despite the severity of the bleeding, my anguish was purely emotional. Tears filled my eyes as I asked, "Why does this keep happening?" But the nurse didn't answer. She just kept wiping up the blood.

After a few minutes that felt like a lifetime, I noticed that the blood flow had subsided. A doctor came in to examine me and said, "Your bleeding has stopped again, but I'm going to ask you to stay in the hospital for seven to ten days for observation. Two severe hemorrhages in a matter of hours are cause for concern."

Seven to ten days! Joe and I looked at each other. Was this really how I was going to spend the next week—hooked up to an IV and stuck in a hospital bed with ultrasound equipment wrapped around me, nurses taking my blood pressure every few hours, separated from my five-year-old?

Joe didn't miss a beat as his tenacity kicked in. "I will handle getting Angelina to and from school," he said. "It's only a week. We have friends and family close by. We'll take care of it. You'll be out of here in no time."

I nodded and thanked him, but I felt hollowed out. For my entire pregnancy, I had prayed every night before bed that I would give birth to happy and healthy babies. It was the best way I knew to mitigate my prenatal anxiety. Now, I had to wonder if my prayers were getting through at all.

As that cold Saturday morning stretched into afternoon, I kept placing my hands on my belly to reassure myself that the twins were still in there. I felt my boy snuggling near my hips. My girl hung out under my ribs, active as usual. I could recognize them already by movement alone. I also wondered about Angelina—how she was doing with my parents, whether she was worried at all, when I could speak with her, and how long I would have to go without seeing her.

Joe and I sat together quietly. We talked a bit, called our families to update them, looked at the TV, looked out the window, looked at each other. If anyone had peeked into the room, we would have appeared calm, but inside each of us was a bubbling cauldron threatening to overflow.

When Joe began pacing from one end of the room to the other, the doctor said, "It looks like Jenny's doing okay for now. If you want to grab some food or take a break, this is the time to do it."

Joe nodded. "Thanks, Doc." He turned to me and said, "I'm going to go downstairs to get something to eat. Would you like anything?"

"No, I'm okay," I said. "See you soon."

As Joe and the doctor disappeared through the doorway, my unanswerable questions came rushing back: *Why does this keep happening? Are my babies in danger? Am I in danger?*

As if my body were reading my mind, it happened again. This time, the third time, was the worst of all. This time, I could feel the blood streaming, pouring, cascading out of me. I felt like I was losing every drop of blood I had, and it wasn't stopping.

I let out a stifled sob. "Nurse!" I yelled, pushing the call button frantically again.

Two nurses rushed in and went about their tasks with laser focus. The large, rectangular gauze pads beneath me, like the kind used to house-train puppies, were soaked through and bright red. Grabbing them from under my legs, one nurse placed them quickly on the scale to measure the amount of blood I had lost. Her face was grim as she read the numbers.

While the second nurse slid fresh pads underneath me, I grabbed my phone and texted Joe: *Come upstairs, now!*

More hospital staff joined the first two nurses, and the doctors began conversing with them in low tones. I could still hear my babies' heartbeats, but they seemed to be changing tone, getting slower... and slower... and slower... And as their cadence changed, so did my alertness. I had lost so much blood by then that I was beginning to feel dizzy and drowsy. My vision started tunneling, threatening to take me down into complete blackness.

I had the distant thought, *Where is Joe? Why is he taking so long to get here?* In reality, he had been gone only minutes.

Just as I was wondering if I would lose consciousness before he came back, one of the nurses leaned over me, speaking close to my face. "Looks like you're going to have these babies today," she said as I sat with a blank stare, trying to process what I had just heard. "But don't worry—we've got this, girl. This place is a well-oiled machine!" she continued.

Is it, though? I wondered. Suddenly, I couldn't breathe. I couldn't think. I couldn't focus on anything besides the certainty that my body was shutting down and the fate of our survival was in someone else's hands.

CHAPTER 4

Fade to Black

_____

I had just stepped out of Jenny's room for the much-needed breather that the doctor had suggested. As I waited for the elevator, I thought, *Shit. I can't believe this is happening.* I had made a point of remaining calm in front of my wife—the last thing she needed was to see me panicking when she was potentially fighting both for her life and for our unborn twins' lives—but I had no playbook for a situation like this.

I took several deep breaths, reminding myself of all the positives in the scenario: *Okay, the babies are fine. If Jenny has to stay in bed for two weeks or three weeks or a month, then that's what she's going to do, because the most important thing is to keep those babies in there as long as possible.* By the time I got off the elevator on the hospital's ground floor, I had convinced myself that everything was under control. I just needed to take care of some logistics.

I had a few phone calls to make. First, I dialed my house. When my mother-in-law answered, I gave her an update on Jenny and the twins. I did not want to over worry her, so I kept my voice neutral as I said, "For now, she's stable and everything seems okay, but she's probably going to have to stay here for a week. Let me figure out the details, and then I'll let you know if we need more help." Thankfully, Jenny's parents had returned from a trip overseas the night before, just in time to be here for what had now transpired. I couldn't imagine if I'd had to deliver this news about their daughter and unborn grandchildren while they were oceans away.

After we spoke, I asked to talk to Angelina. I wanted to explain to her that Mommy and Daddy were at the doctor's but that we would be home soon. I wanted her to hear my voice—and I wanted to hear hers just as much.

"Hi, baby girl. How are you doing?" I asked.

"Good! Me and Vovó are playing UNO, and I beat her five times!" Vovó and Vô are what we call Grandma and Grandpa in Portuguese.

"That's great, honey. I'm glad you're having fun. Mommy and the babies are resting, but she sends lots of kisses."

"Okay, Daddy. Give Mommy a hug for me. Bye," Angelina said in her innocent voice.

After I hung up, I called my sister and then my brothers-in-law to fill them in as well. My sister's house was only five miles away from ours, and Jenny's two older brothers, with whom she was very close, lived two hours away. They immediately wanted to make the drive, but I knew we didn't need any more factors heightening the anxiety in Jenny's room, so I reassured them that everything was going to be okay. "This is not an emergency," I said. "I really don't think you guys need to come right now; I just wanted you to be aware of the situation. I'll call you again at the end of the day."

"Okay," they said. "Just let us know if anything changes or if you need anything."

Strolling across the courtyard to grab a bite, I made my final call, to my best friend since sixth grade. He was Portuguese American too, the best man in my wedding, future godfather to my son, and our wives and children were now close friends. He was the person I always reached out to in times of trauma.

"Hey, man," I began.

As soon as I finished telling him everything that had happened in the past 12 hours, he said, "I'm so sorry. I'm on my way to the hospital right now."

"No, no, no, we're going to be fine," I said. "Jenny just needs to rest right now. We need to keep those babies inside her for as long as we can so that we can get them as close to their due date as possible." It was only January. The twins' due date, May 2, felt so far away.

I got in line at the hospital café as I continued talking to him, tapping my fingers rapidly on the glass display case in front of me. As the smell of fresh pastries filled my nostrils, my stomach started growling. I hadn't realized how hungry I was.

Just as I was retrieving my order, my phone pinged with a text from Jenny.

"Uh, hey, man, I gotta…" I hung up mid-sentence, shoved the phone into my pocket, and ran out of the café, leaving my food behind.

When I exited the elevator on Jenny's floor, I looked toward her room at the end of the hallway. As an orthopedic medical device representative, I attended surgeries every day. I was no stranger to this hospital. Yet, as I glimpsed the havoc outside her door, the whole environment felt foreign to me. I felt as if the sinister music that starts right before something terrible happens in a movie had just begun to play. In a flash, I was sprinting down the hall.

People were rushing in and out, lights were blinking, alarms were sounding, and doctors were screaming orders. I watched helplessly as the nurses pulled blood-soaked pads and towels out from under Jenny's small body.

My breath caught in my throat. I choked out questions: "What's going on? Is she going to be okay?"

I wasn't sure if anyone had heard me until a nurse took me aside. "Jenny is bleeding severely again," she said. "We need to get her a blood transfusion and take her to the operating room immediately. These babies need to come out now."

As she shoved consent forms and a pen at me, my hands shook. I could see a nurse trying to get a blood transfusion going, prepping the lines with saline, making sure there were no bubbles inside. Medical terminology floated around me:

Some of the injections were corticosteroids to help the babies' lungs mature before being born. Others were to prep Jenny for surgery. I didn't understand it all, but I had no trouble grasping the urgency with which the doctors and nurses were working to save my wife and my unborn children. As they whirled around the room in a choreographed ballet that they had no doubt danced hundreds of times before, that realization still did not assure me that my wife and our twins would be safe. Every hypothetical scenario played out in my head: *What if she doesn't make it? What if the babies don't make it?*

This was something I couldn't fix after all. My mind quickly focused on one thing: getting to Jenny's side. I tried to approach her, but it was impossible—she was surrounded by medical personnel. When I finally caught a glimpse of her face, I could tell she was getting weaker by the second. Her half-closed eyes gazed at the ceiling, as if the world around her had stopped. I knew my world would end too if she didn't survive.

The nurses grabbed hold of the sides of Jenny's bed and rolled her out of the room. I quickly followed, grabbing Jenny's hand as we raced down the hall. The walls whirred by me at hyperspeed, white and tan, sterile and empty.

"Everything's going to be okay," I said to Jenny. "Hang in there." I wondered if she was fully there. Could she even see or hear me? Would she remember this later?

As the hospital bed clattered through a set of double doors, one of the nurses pointed to a small room on my left and said, "All right, Dad, you're going to have to stay here."

"I want to be in there with my wife," I said. "I'm credentialed. I'm in the OR every day for work."

"We need to get scrubs for you," the nurse said. "We'll be back for you once we have everything. Just hold tight here."

Hold tight? How can I hold tight and stay back in a moment like this? As the staff prepared to commence their journey to the OR, Jenny looked directly at me for one instant. "Take care of Angelina," she whispered.

When I heard my wife's voice, my stomach dropped.

No. Is she giving up? Does she think it's all over?

"Things will be okay, Jen," I said. "I promise."

She didn't respond. Her distant stare returned. She could barely keep her eyes open. I watched as they slowly fluttered shut.

CHAPTER 5

Expecting the Unexpected

Angelina's green eyes were squeezed tightly closed as she sat up in her bed. She clasped her hands together as she repeated the same prayer she said every night: She wanted nothing more than a baby brother *and* sister. Not one sibling, but two.

"Dear Lord, could you please help me get a baby brother and a baby sister? I promise to be the best big sister I can be."

"Why do you want two babies?" I asked, chuckling. "Is it because you have cousins who are twins?" My brother had fraternal twins, a boy and a girl, close to Angelina's age, and she lived for playing with them and her other cousins. She cherished every holiday at Vovó's—racing around the house, playing tag or hide-and-seek while eating all the delicious food and fresh bread that Vovó stayed up all night preparing, waiting for Santa to show up at the front door on Christmas Eve.

"No," Angelina said, giggling. "I just can't decide between a brother and a sister, so I want one of each!"

I had no doubt that she would be the most loving big sister any younger sibling could dream of. She was the epitome of a good kid. An innocent, sweet, and kind soul. A little girl who always said "please" and "thank you." A well-rounded, creative, active child who kept the three of us busy with gymnastics, dancing, swimming, and her obsession with art. Joe and I wanted nothing more than to make her happy.

"Well, I guess we'll see what happens," I said as I tucked her into bed.

"Okay." She smiled up at me.

Joe and I had already long been trying for another baby. Family was important to all of us. It was in our blood—part of our shared Portuguese culture. The fact that Angelina wanted to have a big family of her own made Joe and me want it even more. But we soon realized that even one additional baby would be a nearly impossible feat for us. Although we had no diagnosed infertility issues, we couldn't seem to succeed at answering our daughter's prayers, despite her undying positivity and unwavering faith.

Then, finally, after months of whiplash between hope and disappointment, I missed my cycle and took a pregnancy test that was positive. At seven weeks, the internet said the baby was the size of a blueberry and that its tiny arms were already noticeable.

One day at work, I took a restroom break, stretching my legs after hours of sitting at my desk. Suddenly, I felt a large clump of something slide out of my body. I checked beneath me and froze when I saw a blood clot sitting at the bottom of the toilet bowl.

I quickly visited my OB, who confirmed my worst fear. "Yes, you miscarried," she said.

I didn't know how I was supposed to make sense of the news, or how I would cope with the sadness. I knew only that I had to keep trying.

After a year had passed, I got pregnant again, but this time, I didn't get my hopes up too much. Even though the pregnancy seemed to be progressing, we couldn't be sure until my first ultrasound that the baby was growing.

On the day of that appointment, Joe took time off work to go with me to the clinic. I held my breath in the dark exam room while we waited for the ultrasound tech to arrive.

As the tech moved a wand in firm circles across my belly, we watched patiently while the usual grainy patterns and strange black caverns took shape on the screen above us. Even though I had seen similar images many times when I was pregnant with Angelina, it was hard to make out what we were seeing. The tech paused periodically to take screenshots and measurements. Suddenly, she hung up the wand on its bracket and said, "I need to get the doctor. We'll be with you in just a minute."

"Is something wrong?" I asked. My heart began to pound. *Oh, no*, I thought. *I can't be having another miscarriage.*

Please, not again. I felt my lips trembling as I tried not to cry.

"The doctor will explain everything," the tech said.

When the doctor entered the room, he didn't look like someone who was about to deliver a death sentence. On the contrary, shortly after he resumed examining me with the ultrasound wand, he said, "Congratulations!"

For what? I wondered.

"There are two," he continued.

"Two *what?*" Joe said.

"Two heartbeats," the doctor said, smiling,

My mouth fell open as my mind erected a stone wall in front of his words. I stared at him as though I hadn't heard him.

"Yes, there are definitely two," he repeated into the silence.

"Are you kidding me?" Joe asked. I couldn't even look at him.

"No, sir. We don't joke about twins," the doctor said. "This right here is Baby A." He turned the volume up so we could hear the surging heartbeat of our first baby. Navigating to the other side of my stomach, he showed us another dark spot with a pattering heart. "And this is Baby B."

What?! I screamed internally, in complete surprise. The heartbeats might as well have been a drum corps, the sound seemed so amplified in the small space. When I finally got up the courage to glance over at Joe, his face was blank, but I could see the wheels churning in his head. *He's flipping out—I know he is*, I thought.

The doctor cleared his throat. "I'll give you two a moment alone. It's normal to experience this news as a shock. Why don't you get dressed and then meet with our patient coordinator?"

After he stepped out of the room, I got dressed quickly and silently, then a nurse escorted Joe and me to a brightly lit office a few doors down the hall. The woman waiting there smiled as she slid a bundle of pamphlets across the desk to us. "I know you weren't expecting this," she said, "but here's some information that might help you prepare for a pregnancy with twins. And if you have any questions, feel free to reach out to us."

I have so many questions. Where do I even begin? I thought, as I mutely accepted the papers from her.

Joe and I were still in utter shock as we walked out to the clinic's parking lot. Neither of us had planned to take a full day off work. After all, having twins didn't actually count as an emergency. We gave each other a long-drawn-out hug. "Let's let this news settle and we can talk about it later. See you at home?" I said to him, heading to my car.

"See you there," he said, unlocking his.

As I drove back to my office, I thought about Joe. If I knew him, his mind would be racing at one hundred miles per hour and he would be blasting music in his car in an attempt to clear his head before he had to collect himself and face his coworkers. For my part, I already felt the problem solver in me kicking in, alongside my maternal instincts. *We're just going to have to figure this out, So what if it's two babies and not one?*

An extra miracle, I told myself. *They're our babies, no matter what, and we will make it work.*

That night, after we had put Angelina to bed, we sat down in our living room and finally had a real conversation.

"This is so crazy! Do you realize what this means?" Joe's voice shook as he spoke. "Double the crying! Double the diapers and wipes; double the cribs and car seats and bottles and clothes! We'll probably need to get a bigger car. We don't even have enough bedrooms for two more kids, and eventually we'll need a bigger house! They'll have to share a room, and how are they ever going to sleep? As soon as one starts crying, the other will wake up! Don't you remember how hard one baby was? How in the world are we going to handle two newborns and a five-year-old?"

I sighed. I knew he wasn't wrong; I remembered the early days of parenting even one child all too well. Trying to bathe a slippery, screaming newborn before she wiggled out of my hands. Coaxing a crying, desperate newborn to sleep. Or nurturing a crying baby in the middle of the night when all I wanted to do was go back to bed. I couldn't imagine how I would accomplish all of these tasks two times over. Not to mention a kindergartener who'd had my undivided attention for the last five years. Although Angelina had been praying for twins, the reality might be different for her, and I wondered how she'd feel when she was no longer the center of attention.

"It's not going to be easy," I said. "That's for sure. Instead of one blessing, we're fortunate enough to get two blessings.

We're just going to have to work it all out, emotionally, physically, and financially. And just think—we'll have extra snuggles, extra kisses, and more love than we'll know what to do with."

"Besides," I went on, unable to stop the eternal optimist in me from shining through, "think of Angelina. This is exactly what she's been praying for. Imagining the delight on our little girl's face when we tell her she's going to be a big sister to *two* babies makes me smile. Maybe it's not what we were expecting, but just think how wonderful our life will be as a family of five."

CHAPTER 6

Baby A and Baby B

While I waited for the nurse to come back and escort me into the OR, I tried to take comfort in the familiar tasks—putting on scrubs and washing my hands profusely—that I did every day before I attended surgeries for my job. But today was anything but typical. This was my family. And I couldn't imagine what I'd say to Angelina if her mother, brother, and sister didn't make it home.

Alone in the locker room, I lost all feeling in my legs and fell to my knees. All I could think to do was pray. "God, please save Jenny and our babies," I begged, my forehead tense with concentration. "I need them. Angelina needs them. You can't take them away from me now. Please save all three, and I will never doubt your presence in my life. I promise I will be a better man."

As I was finishing my plea, the nurse walked in and said, "Joe, you may come in now. Things are moving fast, so we'll have to hurry."

I felt my adrenaline spiking again while I finished changing and followed the nurse out of the locker room. When I entered the OR, I squinted in the bright lights. As my vision adjusted, I took in the chaotic scene around me. To my right, I saw warm blankets, a shiny steel table full of medical instruments, and oxygen equipment, ready to pump air into our babies' tiny lungs. Four neonatal nurses stood by two enclosed incubators, waiting to administer whatever triage they would need to do.

To my left, Jenny was receiving a transfusion. Ruby-red blood dripped through a tube into her arm. A blue drape covered her lower body. A nurse, an anesthesiologist, a resident, two assistants, and an obstetrician stood around her feet, preparing her for an emergency C-section. She had been having light contractions before her most recent hemorrhage, but there was no time for her to proceed through natural labor. If the babies were to have any chance of survival, her surgical team would have to get them out right away.

As I pressed my fingertips to my throbbing head, a nurse touched my arm and pointed at a small stool near Jenny's left shoulder. "Come," she said, "you can sit there and hold your wife's hand."

Jenny lay on the bed, barely conscious. She kept her eyes closed as the hospital staff toyed with her like a ragdoll.

A nurse abruptly flipped her onto her right side so that the anesthesiologist could initiate a spinal tap. Then they flipped her back over.

Within minutes, they were cutting her open. I squeezed her hand tightly and channeled all my focus into helping her endure the ordeal. No time was wasted.

Past the blue drape, I could see the first baby being pulled out. "Baby A," someone said.

"Congratulations—it's a boy!" the doctor said, holding our son in his palm.

But it didn't feel like a victory at that moment. Our son neither moved nor cried. In the deafening silence, I went numb again. How could the doctor be so cheerful when this tiny being was nearly lifeless?

I wanted to hold him, but I knew he needed immediate care. The doctor handed him over to a nurse, who slipped his torso into a plastic sleeve, slid a tube down his throat, laid him in one of the incubators, and began to place wires all over his frail body.

I didn't want to look away, but the commotion around Jenny reminded me that we weren't finished yet.

"And here's your girl!" the doctor said as Baby B emerged.

One of the nurses took our daughter from him, wrapped her tightly in a warm blanket, and carried her to the second incubator. Unlike her brother, though, my daughter was ready to make her presence known. As a tiny cry escaped her lips, one of the nurses summoned me over. "Did you hear that?" she said.

It sounded more like a squeal to me, but I took out my phone and made a short video. I wanted to include both babies in it, but the nurses were still working on my son. Everything was happening so fast; it was hard to capture every moment.

As I studied the twins—their veins pulsing beneath their translucent skin, their arms and legs like twigs that the slightest pressure could have snapped in half—they didn't look anything like any newborn I had ever seen, including their big sister. Yet here they were, out in the world, and now we and everyone else in the room were united in the common purpose of keeping them alive.

I returned to Jenny's side and put my hand on her shoulder, but she lay still. Even with the transfusion, she had lost too much blood to be responsive. However, when the doctor said, "We need to get these babies to the NICU right away. Dad, you should go with them," I looked at Jenny and she nodded and whispered, "Go. I'll be fine."

"Okay." I kissed her on her forehead and followed the nurses wheeling the two incubators out of the room. While we walked, they acted like we were on our way to a party, not an intensive care unit. "Congratulations, Dad! These babies are beautiful!" they said, beaming at me. I know now that they did this with all parents of preemies, who are likely to have a negative mindset because of the shock they've just experienced and the risks involved in early births, but at the time I just wanted them to stop talking to me so that I could think. *Two days ago, I was trying to figure out how we were going to take care of twins due in May. Now they're four months early and we don't even know if they're going to survive for the next 24 hours. Will I ever even get to hold them?* And Jenny—I could only imagine what was going through her head as she lay alone, barely conscious and just out of a major surgery she never thought she was going to have.

The fact that our hospital had a Level IV NICU, which offers the highest possible level of medical care to newborn and premature infants, was barely enough to slow my thundering heart. To distract myself, I studied the twins' little pods as I walked alongside them.

Baby A: 2 pounds, 0 ounces, 14 inches, read the label on my baby boy's incubator.

Baby B: 1 pound, 11 ounces, 12 inches. My baby girl weighed as much as a loaf of bread and was practically the size of a Barbie doll.

I recalled holding Angelina when she was born, at five pounds, seven ounces, and thinking how small her fingers and toes were, but on these babies, they were unimaginable. That didn't stop me from believing my children were little warriors who would fight through this, though. After all, they had their parents' blood, strength, and willpower.

My racing mind outpacing my footsteps, I followed the nurses into the NICU. They led me into a big room that looked like the inside of a spaceship. They wheeled my son to one side and my daughter to the other and started wiring them up to machines. At some point, one of the nurses said, "Dad, do you want us to take a picture of you with the babies?"

I obliged, but my smile in the photos from that day belies what I was actually thinking in that moment: *I don't know how I haven't passed out yet.*

A few minutes later, the twins' neonatologist came in. He examined them, gave me a nod, and said, "I'll come back in a little while, once I know more."

After he left, I sat in the darkness in a green plastic recliner between the incubators, staring blankly at all the machines in the room and listening to their beeps and clicks. I had lost control of situations in the past, but those events were mild tremors compared to my current earthquake of despair.

After my turbulent childhood and adolescence with my warring parents, I became a young, wild soul in my early twenties. My focus was far from going to college and getting a degree, yet I still had a strong work ethic and an unexpected career ambition. I became a successful real estate agent and began to invest all my money in residential real estate, where my returns were so good that I had cash to burn and spent it on motorcycles, cars, and other recreational pastimes.

By the time I met Jenny in 2007 through a mutual friend, my good fortune had taken a turn for the worse. My cousin, best friend, and mentor was dying of cancer at the young age of 36; my parents were moving back to Portugal; and the real estate market was crashing and left me financially in the hole. At first, I liquidated all my assets and drained my savings account to stay afloat, but eventually I had no choice but to file for bankruptcy.

When I admitted to Jenny that I had lost everything, I was sure she was going to leave me. In fact, I encouraged her to, saying, "I can't drag you into this kind of stress. You deserve better." When that didn't work, I started acting like a jerk, trying to push her away. But she didn't take the bait then either. Against all odds, she saw the permanent potential in me beyond the temporary state of crisis I was in. She paid my bankruptcy attorney's fees. She was always available to listen. She was the first and only woman I ever cried in front of. She helped me to control my lifelong temper and to handle the challenges my parents presented. And she taught me how to be more "me," rather than allowing me to maintain the facade of bravado that I had been wearing for years. Other people whom I thought were my friends had ditched me at the first signs of trouble. Not Jenny—she seemed to have come into my life for the specific purpose of giving me the deep love and support I had always needed. With her encouragement, I found the courage and the motivation to start rebuilding my career, and ultimately to become a better man, husband, father, and entrepreneur.

However, because it wasn't the right time to be a realtor, I leveraged my longtime sales background, which included hospitality and construction, to find a new job. When a real estate teammate of mine, and a longtime friend, recruited me to become a medical device rep specializing in foot and ankle products, I regained my professional footing. Two years later, Jenny and I got married, and finally, Angelina, our first pride and joy, was born.

Now, as I sat in the NICU with my babies, all of my past hurdles seemed inconsequential compared with the catastrophe I was facing today. But I knew Jenny wasn't going to save me this time; she needed to focus on her own recovery so that she could stand by my side for the long journey ahead of us. *Get it together, Joe,* I told myself. *These precious babies need you, and so do Jenny and Angelina.* I straightened a little in my chair, took a deep breath, and silently promised my family that I would never stop fighting for them.

CHAPTER 7

The Calm Before the Storm

For the first few months of my pregnancy, although my belly grew faster than it had with Angelina, not much else was different. I worked, I cooked, I cleaned, and I kept up with Angelina's daily activities. My life was calm, safe, stable, and predictable—just as it had always been.

I have always loved the strength of my culture, and I have always lived in a flurry of joyful tradition. Every summer growing up, my parents, my siblings, and I flew from our hometown in Virginia to Portugal and visited the small villages in the North where my parents were born.

The nearest city, Chaves, is nestled in the mountains near Spain. In my grandparents' farming villages, gray-green olive leaves rustled in the sunshine, creating playful shadows on the cobblestone ground beneath them. Grapes hung in the vineyards, glowing deep red in the evening light. In the barnyard, I played with calves, chickens, and rabbits. I slid my fingers through lambs' rough curls, picking pieces of hay out of them. Their soft pink noses nuzzled mine as I bottle-fed them their milk.

My grandparents made their own wine and olive oil and grew their own vegetables. My brothers and I helped dig for potatoes in their yard, piling them in wood pallets in the stone barn. My grandfather let us ride his donkey and accompany him on the tractor all the way to the high hills to water his vines. We helped him stomp on the grapes, our legs turning purple, and spent long summer afternoons hiking in the mountains and swimming in the rivers. I treasured every life lesson I learned from those idyllic trips to my homeland.

My parents were young teenagers when each of their families immigrated to the United States, settling in Jamaica, New York. My grandmothers were dressmakers in clothing factories and both of my grandfathers worked construction. My mother and father met at a Portuguese dance in their early twenties. She was shy and quiet, one of three sisters who were renowned for their beauty within the local Portuguese community, and he was outgoing, the life of the party. Once they started dating, it wasn't long before they were married and having children. They relocated to Long Island, where my father had his own construction business and where my three brothers and sister were born. I was born in Virginia, where they moved for my father's job.

Although they had come to the United States in search of a better life, my parents still had strong family values and modeled a strong marriage and a loving home. My parents followed the old-school tradition of the father working day and night to provide for the family while the mother stayed home, cleaning, cooking, and watching the children. Life wasn't easy for them in the early stages of their marriage. Before I was even born, they experienced a parent's worst nightmare two times over— the loss of two children, both in hospitals— my sister as a newborn and my brother at the age of three. I always looked up to my parents for being able to pull through all the traumatic events they had to endure. They still managed to sustain a marriage and keep their family together. Even after living through those experiences, I was still brought into this world.

When I was growing up, my parents' room was my favorite place in the house. Its shiny wood floors and eight-foot mirror were irresistible to me, especially when I had time there alone with my mother. I would let out a deep, satisfied sigh whenever her fingers began tenderly brushing my long hair. She helped me choose outfits and clucked her approval while I tried on her makeup, scarves, and jewelry. During thunderstorms, I would lie on the rug by her bed, wanting to be as near to her as possible.

Our kitchen, the site of countless gatherings, delicious meals, and holiday festivities, was another place that spoke to me of happiness and security. My cousins from next door, other relatives, my brothers, and my parents would gather around the large island, feasting on traditional Portuguese food while soccer games played on the TV in the background. We ate delicate codfish filets, roasted octopus tentacles curled among beds of vegetables, succulent lamb, homemade sausages, artisanal cheeses, and fresh homemade bread.

In our living room, the flames in the fireplace crackled as my father sat peacefully on his recliner, television remote in hand. He was a man of respect, dignity, and honor, yet could fill a room with laughter at the slightest joke or smirking remark. When the power went out during winter storms, he and my mother didn't miss a beat in cooking over the fire, honoring our heritage while the aromas of our dinner filled the room. My father took pride in his home—a home that he managed the design and construction of and was always proud of.

My brothers took their jobs as older siblings seriously and always protected me from any harm that might come my way—as well as some opportunities with boys at school who liked me. Everyone knew our family—not just my brothers but also my five male cousins who all lived nearby and were close in age—and no one dared to mess with me. Anytime a boy even tried to spend time with me, one of my relatives would say, "If you break her heart, I'll hurt you." My parents also kept me on a short leash and let me attend high school events like parties and football games only if one of my older brothers was there to chaperone me.

It's a wonder that Joe was able to break through that wall of protection. He had played soccer with my brothers, and he knew that our culture would require him to be respectful of a nice girl from a good home. The first time we met was three years before we started dating, but he knew better than to approach me at the time, when he was still partying and dating up a storm. By the time we actually got together, he was ready to be in a committed relationship. Four years later, I married the husband I had always dreamed of having, and then I became a mother for the first time.

Joe and I took Angelina to Portugal a few times in her first five years of life. We visited Joe's parents and extended family in his hometown and showed her the small towns where both sets of her grandparents grew up. We would take her to see the tiny houses made of stone with no electricity where her grandparents were born. She got to meet her cousins, who did not speak English but found their own ways of communicating with her through dance and play.

Angelina would stand in the doorways of my parents' childhood homes, staring out over the grassy hills and fields of olive trees. She loved Portuguese festivals—a flurry of sequins, flowers, bright traditional outfits, food, music, fireworks, and dancing—as much as I did. These trips not only allowed her to experience the beauty of our home country but also taught her the importance of deep roots and familial bonds.

I couldn't wait to tell Angelina about her new siblings. Twins run in our family. My grandmother had twins and believed that tendency would skip a generation. She always predicted that I would have them too, but, despite her conviction,

I never thought it would be possible. Apparently, Angelina knew something I didn't, because her prayers were going to come true.

On the day Joe and I were to tell her the news, I wrapped special gifts for her in a box tied with a pretty bow. Seated beside her on the couch, I handed the box to her. She held it for a moment before untying the ribbon and opening it. She carefully removed two pacifiers, two bibs, two bottles, and two stuffed animals.

"Are these for my dolls?" she asked.

"Nope," I said. Joe's and my smiles couldn't conceal our excitement.

She paused. "Does… Is this for a baby?" she asked. "Are you having a *baby*?"

When we nodded, Angelina screeched and leaped off the couch. While she jumped and danced around the living room, I asked, "Why do you think there are two of everything in the box?"

She could barely stop jumping, but she paused to give my question some thought. Then she screamed, "Oh my gosh! We're getting *two* babies?"

On that beautiful fall day, our five-year-old daughter raced around the house, wild with joy.

CHAPTER 8

The Recovery Room

I sat in the recovery room, unable to move, repainting the pictures of what had just happened to me. All I could remember were blinding lights, loud noises, and bodies moving all around me while doctors and nurses shouted at each other. I remembered that my son had gone straight into his incubator to be intubated and my daughter had shown at least some sort of life by letting out a tiny squeal. Before they put her in her own incubator, one of the nurses had held her up to my face for a split second while Joe snapped a photo, but I could hardly remember what she looked like. Unfortunately, for me it was all a blur.

It seemed impossible that I had been at work 24 hours earlier, feeling fine and unconcerned about the light spotting

I had experienced over the past week, or even that only one hour earlier I had thought my babies were going to stay inside my body while I spent a week or so in the hospital. I had no knowledge of NICUs and no frame of reference for this experience. My only other pregnancy had been healthy, uneventful, and full-term. *Why did this have to happen so soon?* I asked myself, as a tear slid down my cheek. *Are my babies going to be okay? They don't deserve this.*

I couldn't help but wonder if I was to blame. The cycle of anxiety and doubt that had started earlier in my pregnancy reared up again. *What if my body was too small to carry twins? What if the ultrasound probe I'd had the day before had irritated my uterus and caused irreversible damage? What if that time I fell in the sand at the beach a few weeks prior sent me into preterm labor? What if, what if, what if?* But I had to erase those thoughts from my head and move forward. I had to think positively. Logically, I knew there was nothing I could have done differently.

Meanwhile, Joe was on the move. He had quickly gotten into a frantic routine, spending his time checking on the twins in the NICU, reporting back to me, communicating with his colleagues, attending orthopedic surgeries for work, going home to see Angelina and our dog, Sky, and taking college courses online to fulfill the credits he needed to complete his bachelor's degree. He was running on pure adrenaline, but he managed to do it all. He seemed to have enough energy for both of us.

Whenever he showed up in my room, I had to strain to ask, "How are they?" I could still hardly move, and all the medication I was on made me constantly drowsy.

He always gave me a detailed report. "They're stable, and their temperatures are normal—no infections so far. The doctors say these first few days are critical. The babies are having all kinds of tests: daily bloodwork, X-rays, and head ultrasounds to check for brain bleeds. We need to take it day by day, hour by hour. Things could change at any moment, but for now they're doing okay. They each have their own nurse, who will rotate out every 12 hours, and everyone is so gentle with them. It's amazing how they handle infants this small."

I smiled weakly. It was the least I could do when I knew Joe was trying to keep the mood light. "Do you want to look at the photos I sent?" he asked.

On my phone, I swiped through the images Joe had sent me of the twins immediately after their birth. I could see the babies' arteries and veins showing through their translucent skin. Their eyes were shielded with tape and masks so the NICU lights would not damage them. I could barely make out their facial features under the oxygen masks and tubes covering their faces. Their fingers and toes were mere dots on the screen.

Of course I wanted to see my newborn children, but until I saw those pictures, I had mostly been able to keep up a positive front about their condition: *They're going to be fine; they have the best care we could ever imagine. We are exactly where we need to be, given the circumstances.* I had no idea that the aftermath would be so dire, that I would almost not be able to recognize my babies' features underneath all the tubes and wires and wrappings. I was so concerned about what would happen to me during all the bleeding that the possibility of having one-and two-pound babies didn't even occur to me.

Through all that mess, I knew my son and daughter were beautiful, but these photos were all I had of them. We had had no skin-to-skin bonding as they searched for their first meal. No first family portraits immediately after their delivery. No exhausted triumph as I held one twin in each arm moments after birth. What should have been a precious moment for all of us had been taken away forever.

I knew Joe didn't want to dwell on these losses any more than I did. Sensing my distress as I scrutinized the pictures, he changed the subject. "Any ideas about names?" he asked. "They can't be Baby A and Baby B forever."

We had brainstormed a few times and narrowed down the list to a few names, but we were far from making our final decision. "I can't even see their faces in these photos," I said. "To be honest, they don't even look real. How are we supposed to name them?"

Joe shrugged. "How about Alyssa, Gabriella, or Layla?"

I shook my head.

"Luke, Luca, or Jackson?"

I didn't know.

"This is so hard!" I said, fighting pain and exhaustion.

"Maybe Angelina can help us decide when she visits," Joe offered.

"Yes, let's ask her. I think she'd like that," I said, falling back on my pillow. "She'll know."

Later that evening, the nurse told me there was one thing I could do to help my babies: begin pumping every three hours so they could begin to get my breastmilk.

She set the pump on the table beside my bed. "You probably remember from your first delivery that colostrum is the yellow milk that your body produces in the first few days after your babies are born. It's filled with powerful nutrients. That's why we call it liquid gold. When you go visit your babies, you can put a drop at a time on their tongues using a Q-Tip. You'll be surprised how quickly their instincts kick in."

"Of course! I can do that." I smiled genuinely for what felt like the first time in weeks. After constantly feeling numb and powerless, finally, something was in my control. Finally, I might actually be able to help.

"How are they getting nutrients now?" I asked.

"Right now, they're being given TPN, total parenteral nutrition, through an umbilical catheter, which will deliver essential nutrients and minerals through their veins and all the way to the heart. Soon, they will receive a PICC line, or a peripherally inserted central catheter, and eventually, once they're ready, we'll begin giving them your breastmilk through a feeding tube, supplementing whatever you can't produce with donor breastmilk. Right now, their digestive tract is not mature enough to take in milk, but it's best we start stocking up now.

All afternoon, I threw myself into pumping. *If I'm going to be stuck in this hospital bed, I thought, I'm going to try to be useful and give these kids what they need so they can grow and get better.* After all they had been through, it was the least I could do—not to mention the only thing I could do.

The doctor assured me, "You'll be able to visit the babies as soon as you're strong enough to get out of bed and into a wheelchair on your own. But for now, you need to work hard on healing, resting, eating healthy, and staying hydrated. That will maximize your chances of seeing them as soon as possible."

"I will," I promised.

"You did an amazing job carrying this pregnancy as far as you did. Your babies are in great hands," he added.

After the doctor stepped out into the hall, I took a moment of gratitude for his kindness, and for the fact that my babies and I were all—remarkably—still alive, at least for the time being. But it would be a long time before I would be able to erase the memory of a rush of blood flowing down my legs. I would sometimes wake in a cold sweat and quickly touch the mattress underneath me to confirm that I was okay.

"Are you sure there's no chance I'll bleed again?" I kept asking my nurse.

"You're doing great, honey," she said, for the third time in a single day. "I've checked your uterus, and everything is normal. You have no reason for alarm."

On my second full day in the hospital, I heard a light knock on the door of my room. Angelina walked in with a big smile on her face, my parents and Joe close behind. She hurried over to me and melted into my arms. I couldn't help but notice how enormous she looked compared with her brother and sister.

"Why are you in this bed?" she asked, frowning as she took in my hospital gown and the IV attached to my arm.

I thought for a moment, then decided to keep things simple. "I have to stay in the hospital for a few days," I said. "Check out these special buttons. See? This button makes the bed go up, and this one makes it go down."

Angelina grinned as she pushed the controls for a few seconds, but she had other things on her mind. "Where are my brother and sister?" she asked.

"They're in a special room upstairs for newborns, getting care from lots of great nurses," I said.

"Can I see them? Can I hold them?"

"Not yet, honey," Joe said. As Angelina's face fell, he added, "I know it's hard, baby girl. But your brother and sister came into this world a little sooner than expected, so now the doctors and nurses need to help them get stronger so they can grow. When they do, then you'll be able to see them. In the meantime, we're hoping you can help us pick their names."

At that, Angelina smiled. "Hmm…" She paused, deep in thought.

"What are your thoughts on Gabriella, Alyssa, or Layla for your sister, and Jackson, Luca, or Luke for your brother?"

I asked.

"I like Layla for my sister and Luke for my brother."

"Luke and Layla." I said it out loud. "I love that. Those names sound perfect together." I already knew Joe would approve. I nodded. "It's decided," I said, and gave Angelina a big hug.

I glanced over at my parents to see if they approved, but they seemed too worried to have even heard our conversation.

"Can I go see them?" my mom asked.

"Of course. Joe can take you up there. Dad, do you want to go?"

"No, I'll stay here with you and Angelina," he said. I didn't press him, because I knew he would have joined my mom if he had been ready to handle the sight.

As Joe walked my mom upstairs, I spent some much-needed time with my dad and Angelina, thanking God I was still around to hold her tight.

CHAPTER 9

Don't Google Any-thing

After Angelina and my in-laws left the hospital, I went upstairs to check on the babies again while Jenny took a nap.

The room was dark, the only light coming from the fluorescent bulbs in the electrocardiogram monitors. The only sound was the whisper of what appeared to be forced air coming out of Layla's SiPAP oxygen machine, a noninvasive ventilation system that was supporting her respiratory activity. The prongs inserted in her nostrils were attached to a tube taped to her face on one end and attached to the machine on the other. *The nose prongs look so uncomfortable*, I thought. Luke, meanwhile, was still intubated. The doctor had explained that the babies didn't know how to breathe on their own yet, given their internal organs were so underdeveloped, so the machines helped facilitate the effort.

They were both swaddled tightly, wearing knit caps the size of Post-it notes, sleeping peacefully across the room from each other. Their incubators were set to skin temperature mode at 89.6 degrees Fahrenheit (32 degrees Celsius) to keep their bodies at a similar temperature to the one they had experienced inside the womb, with an added 70 percent humidity for their skin. The nurses had situated them in the fetal position and stuffed rolled-up blankets around their bodies to keep them from moving around. Once in a while, one of them would jerk or twitch a bit, but for the most part they didn't move. Whenever I caught a glimpse of them, I shuddered.

The nurses routinely checked their blood pressure and temperature, pricked their heels for blood to check for signs of infection, and weighed their used diapers to ensure that their digestive tracts were working properly. Electrode lead patches attached to the babies' chests constantly sensed and recorded signals traveling through their hearts. And a pulse oximeter wrapped around their tiny feet measured their oxygen saturation levels.

The thought of the doctors inserting a PICC line into each of their ankles made me cringe. Their arms were no bigger than my finger and their blood vessels were as thin as sewing thread. *How is this procedure even possible?* I wondered. *It's hard enough when my doctor tries to find a vein in me; I can't imagine what it's like doing that on a premature baby.*

While I sat in my usual green chair, I thought about my limited knowledge of twins. I knew most were born at least slightly prematurely and at lower birth weights, but Luke and Layla were anything but typical. Before I could resist, I grabbed my phone and typed "Survival rate of babies born at 26 weeks" into the search bar.

When the statistics popped up, I wanted to look away. The results told me that two out of every ten babies at that age would not survive, and that one out of ten would have serious complications, such as a brain bleed, anemia, learning disabilities, cerebral palsy, sepsis, or loss of vision or hearing. The fact that we had two premature babies versus a singleton made our odds even worse.

A few minutes later, as if he had been looking over my shoulder, the doctor gave me a warning. "Do me a favor. Don't Google anything," he said.

"Uh, it's a little too late, Doc," I said, as I put my phone down. "Let me ask you honestly: What are the chances our babies will survive and live a normal life?"

He stopped looking at the chart he was examining and looked right at me with kind eyes. "Every day is going to be crucial right now," he said. "You've already seen that we're constantly monitoring their essential signs of life and making sure they're not developing any kind of infection. Due to their lack of immune system and the considerable number of invasive procedures they've had, the risk of an infection is a major concern, which is why we have given them antibiotics. Right now, we see no real indications of serious complications, but it's too early to tell what the future holds. Their vital organs are severely underdeveloped, including their lungs, their hearts, and their digestive systems. In addition, we're monitoring their brains to detect any type of brain bleeds. Signs of severe injury usually show up during the first few weeks of life; develop-mental delays could show up later. But there are so many variables at play right now, it's too hard to predict the outcome. Every hour, every day, is a milestone. You're going to feel like you're taking one step forward and then three steps back for the next few months."

"How long do you think they'll be in the NICU?" I asked.

"Probably until their due date, at the very least," the doctor said.

But that's almost four months away, I thought.

When the doctor noticed my downcast face, he said, "No matter what, none of this is your fault or your wife's fault. NICU parents tend to put the blame on themselves. But there is nothing you or Jenny could have done to prevent what happened."

I nodded. "Thanks, Doc."

After he left, I paced the twins' dark room, checking my phone, texting Jenny, and whispering to my babies through their plastic enclosures. I desperately wanted to hold them and tell them everything was going to be okay. But was that the truth? After all, the doctor had just told me there were no guarantees. All Jenny and I could do was take one step forward, three steps back, and pray for the best.

When a beeping alarm interrupted the quiet, I instantly felt my blood pressure rise. Staring helplessly at the flashing numbers on the monitors, I thought, *What is happening?*

A nurse rushed in, poked her hand into Layla's incubator, unwrapped her partially, and nudged her arm. The beeping stopped as suddenly as it had started.

"What just happened?" I asked, holding my chest.

"The monitor alerted me that Layla forgot to breathe," the nurse said. "It's called apnea of prematurity when they stop breathing for a short period of time. The part of our brain that tells us we need to breathe is not developed yet in a micropreemie. Typically, it begins to develop around 34 to 35 weeks' gestation. We just have to poke her gently to wake her and remind her to breathe—that's all. It's apnea and bradycardia, which usually happen together when a baby's breathing stops, triggering a low heart rate. It's very normal in premature babies. You'll get very accustomed to it, as it will happen frequently while they're still so underweight and underdeveloped. We call them 'episodes' or 'As and Bs'. Believe it or not, at this age, we administer doses of caffeine citrate to jump-start their respiratory system. We gave them a large dose when they were first admitted and will continue to give them a dose every 24 hours for the next few weeks."

I wondered how Layla felt. *Is she in any pain? She looks so peaceful—does she have any idea what's happening around her?* I had read that babies can feel pain after 22 weeks.

The nurse didn't look concerned in the slightest. She just shot me a smile, wrote a few numbers on Layla's chart, and left the room. But as soon as she was gone, my whole body tensed up. In that moment, I felt as if somebody had just punched me in my gut. I doubled over in my chair, put my head in my hands, and closed my eyes.

The next thing I knew, I was waking up to the same beeping sound I'd heard before I had dozed off. This time, the nurse started poking at Luke. However, he didn't respond right away like Layla had before. The nurse quickly opened his incubator, picked him up, and removed his swaddle. "Come on, Luke. Wake up, buddy," the nurse said. His tiny, gangly body wiggled as she startled him over and over. His hands jolted violently, and then he started breathing again and the beeping finally stopped. I watched as his oxygen level on the screen rose back to 99 again.

As the machine settled down, I realized I hadn't been breathing during those moments either. I let out a long, tattered sigh. *What happens if they don't get to him quickly enough next time?*

For the rest of the evening shift, the crises and sounds of the alarms bounced back and forth between Luke and Layla like a sick tennis match. First Layla would have an episode and forget to breathe; then, as soon as she seemed okay, Luke would be in distress. It was always something.

How am I going to tell my wife that our babies just stop breathing spontaneously or that their hearts need to be restarted?

I wondered. *No mother should ever have to hear that, let alone a mother who's been through what she's been through.*

But sometimes our only choice is to tell the truth, even when it hurts. *Keep it together, Joe,* I reminded myself. I whispered to the babies that I'd be back soon and anxiously walked out of their room.

day two post-delivery | jenny

CHAPTER 10

The NICU

When word got out that I had delivered my babies, my phone began flooding with text messages and phone calls from family members and friends. It was so hard to respond with the truth when asked how I was doing and if everything was okay.

No, I was not okay, the babies were not okay, and nothing anyone else could do would change that. While I was happy to be alive and that my babies had made it out alive, the combination of our recent trauma and our unknown future was more than I could bear.

Flowers and cards covered my hospital room windowsill, and people seemed more comfortable expressing their concern with such gifts than with words. My brothers drove to visit me as soon as they could, as did many other loved ones, but when I tried to converse with them, I could tell that most of them didn't know what to say or how to act. They would give me quick hugs and stare awkwardly at the babies' photos without saying anything.

Still, I relied heavily on my visitors to lift my spirits during those early days in the hospital. I also had a dedicated social worker who reached out to me by phone on a daily, sometimes hourly, basis. "How are you feeling?" she would ask. "Is there anything I can do to help? Whenever you start to feel down, I'd like you to call me." She seemed like a wonderful resource for mothers in my situation, but mostly I told her, "Obviously I'm not doing great, but I think I'm okay, and thankfully I have a lot of other support." Hashing out what had happened only brought tears to my eyes every time I even thought about it, much less tried to speak about it.

I just wasn't in the right frame of mind to engage much with the outside world beyond my immediate family. I had a singular mission that required all of my focus and energy: to fight for Luke and Layla's health, to keep communicating with Joe, to keep Angelina's life as normal as possible, and ultimately to get all of us back together so we could all move forward.

A day and a half after my C-section, I received clearance to go up to the NICU and visit my newborn babies. I would finally get to see in person everything Joe had been telling me about. Luke and Layla would hear my voice again, the voice they had heard every day in the womb. Even if I couldn't hold them yet, I could be with them and let them hear my voice. And that would be enough for now.

Joe rolled a wheelchair into my room. "Are you ready?" he asked.

"Ready as I'll ever be," I said. "Let's go."

I slid gingerly from my hospital bed into the wheelchair, my heart pounding. We took the elevator up to the NICU floor and were greeted by a host of rules and security precautions that NICU visitors must comply with: taking off all nail polish or jewelry so we wouldn't bring any mold, germs, or infection-causing agents into the area; signing in and receiving approval to enter; and calling the nurses to let them know we were there so they could buzz us through the double doors.

The front-desk staff already knew Joe well. His frequent visits had made him a regular. They buzzed us in immediately. As he wheeled me through the double doors, I secured my ID bracelet around my wrist. When we reached a bank of large sinks and hand-sanitizing stations, Joe said, "Time to lather up. Wash your arms all the way up to your elbows, and don't forget your fingernails. Wash for one minute, and then sanitize right after."

I did as he said while eying the wall clock. One full minute felt like a lifetime, but I couldn't run the risk of transmitting even one life-threatening germ to my babies.

After we sanitized, Joe wheeled me down the hall. The walls were painted in welcoming earth tones, but many of the other parents pacing outside the rooms, their faces wrinkled with worry, looked anything but soothed. As I passed the mothers, some of them locked eyes with me, transmitting the depth of their fears and binding us forever in our shared experience.

Large, framed photos of NICU survivors lined the corridor. A few showed twins who had been born as early as 24 to 26 weeks, while others had made it all the way to 30 or even 32 weeks. Every picture and every triumphant smile had a joyous story to tell—one that no doubt was the result of heroic efforts by the doctors and nurses in this hospital.

These are beautiful, I thought, a glimmer of hope sparking in my heart.

"It's a wall of hope," I whispered to Joe. I closed my eyes for a moment and prayed that images of Luke and Layla would one day hang there to encourage other desperate families.

After reading some of these babies' stories in the photo captions, I was ready to pass through the double doors ahead of me. The central nurses' station was surrounded on all sides by sliding doors that led to the babies' individual rooms. Luke and Layla's room was the first one on the left.

I asked Joe to pause outside their door. It was shut. I felt like I had to catch my breath as I wondered, *How can any of this be real? How can it be true that I'm about to visit my babies in their very own hospital room?*

After a moment, Joe squeezed my shoulder and turned toward the nurses' station to let them know that I was ready to go in. Luke's nurse came over to greet me. "Hi, Mama, it's great to see you. Your babies are beautiful," she said as she slid open the door.

The room was pitch black with fluorescent light accents, just as Joe had described it to me. There was a divider in the center of the room that had been pushed back to make it one large double room for twins. Each side of the room was a mirror image of the other. As my eyes adjusted, I could barely see the babies' temperature-controlled incubators, each covered in a crocheted blanket, one pink and one blue. A steady whirring sound shooed out of the SiPAP oxygen machine.

Glancing around the room, I took in the whiteboards featuring my children's daily charts, listing their nurses' names; their weight and length; and whatever procedures, labs, scans, or X-rays they would have that day. They also listed goals for the babies—something to look forward to or a milestone to work toward. A small refrigerator on the floor held my breastmilk, and two green recliners were waiting for us to sit, sleep, pump, and, I hoped, hold the babies some day. I wondered how many days we would spend practically living inside this room.

I was so nervous, but I needed to get on with it. I had not come here to stare at these unfamiliar surroundings. It was time for me to get out of my wheelchair, hobble over and see my newborns.

"I'm going to get the doctor now that you're finally here," the nurse said, and slipped out.

Since Luke was closest to the door, Joe grabbed my arm and helped me up so I could approach him. I read the sign taped to his incubator stating he was only 2lb, as if to confirm that he was real, and then, taking a deep breath, I lifted the soft crocheted blue blanket that hung on top and peeked inside.

Maybe I had hoped that Luke wouldn't look the same way he had in the pictures, but I couldn't deny the resemblance. His tiny blue hat. His eye mask. His delicate skin. Tubes coming from his nose and mouth. Numerous wires snaking out from under his blanket on all sides.

I couldn't hold back my tears. For the past two days, I had been too shocked and stunned, too focused on being strong, to fully cry. Now, I couldn't suppress my pain any longer. As I realized there was nothing I could do to help my son, I began to sob uncontrollably.

Joe immediately grabbed me and held me tight. We both knew that hope and faith were our only tools for battling the uncertainty our family faced.

Wiping my eyes with my hospital gown, I made my way over to Layla. Her sign told me she was even smaller than Luke. Under her pink blanket, I witnessed a similar scene. She lay on her tummy, totally still, utterly helpless yet somehow deeply peaceful. An oxygen mask covered her nose and she wore a tiny pink hat.

The nurse had said I could touch the babies over their blankets, so I opened the incubator's small, circular door as gently as I could, as if trying not to scare her. Sliding my hand through its narrow opening, I placed my index finger on Layla's forehead. I could have engulfed her entire skull with my hand. Her precious, vein-mapped skin looked so fragile that I was afraid to touch her, but I couldn't help myself. She was still so beautiful.

"Hi, Layla," I whispered. "It's Mommy. I'm so sorry you had to come into this world so early, but you're doing great. Mommy and Daddy love you so much. We're going to be right by your side every day to fight this with you. You will never be alone, and I have faith that you're going to make it through this. Your brother, Luke, is right across the room, fighting with you, and you have a big sister at home who can't wait to meet you."

I walked back over to Luke and said the same things to him as I stroked his finger. I knew it would be days or weeks before I could cradle these babies in my arms, but I needed them to hear my voice. I needed them to know that I was there and that it was going to be okay, even if it wasn't.

It's not supposed to be this way, I thought, bursting into tears again as I slowly took my hand out of Luke's incubator. These two babies, who had snuggled with each other for the past 26 weeks, had been ripped apart from one another and now had to sleep on opposite sides of a room that looked like something out of a sci-fi movie.

Just then, the doctor came in with the nurses. I tried to focus on what he was saying as he delivered a barrage of information.

"I'm glad to see you," he said. "The babies each had to receive a blood transfusion today because their red blood cell counts were low. This will help increase their red blood cell count and prevent anemia. We'll complete their brain scans and continue to take blood tests to detect any infection—one of our biggest concerns at this point. Even a full-term baby's immune system is just kicking in at birth. It takes a while for a premature baby to catch up. In fact, even though they're severely preterm, they will soon receive their first required vaccine to ensure that they stay on the pediatric immunization schedule and undergo the same precautions that full-term infants do."

He paused for a moment, then continued when Joe nodded. "I can't tell you one way or the other how this will go for them, but I can tell you that they're stable and doing great so far. Anything could happen, but we need to just keep hoping that they continue trending in the right direction. All we can do is take things hour by hour."

When the doctor finished talking, Joe thanked him, but I couldn't even speak. I just kept on crying. My babies were missing months of my antibodies and nourishment that would help them fight off disease. Their brains weren't developed enough to tell them when to breathe, and their lungs weren't strong enough to function on their own. I couldn't even hold them.

I buried my head in my hands. *Why did this have to happen?* I wanted nothing more than to cradle Luke and Layla in my arms and protect them from harm. Better yet, I wished I could grab them and stick them back inside my body, where they would be safe.

It was all too much. As hard as it was to leave their sides, I climbed back into my wheelchair and gestured to Joe to take me back to my room.

CHAPTER 11

Empty

On Tuesday, four days after I was admitted to the hospital, I was discharged. *So soon?* I wondered. *Am I actually okay to go home, after everything that's happened?* The idea that I could go back home, sleep in my own bed, and be with Angelina was irresistible, except for the nagging thought that I was now a mother of three and two of those children were still hospitalized. All I wanted was to be in two places at once.

The backseat was empty and the car was quiet as Joe and I pulled out of the hospital parking lot. My mind was racing, yet I couldn't seem to put any of those thoughts into words. We'd been in this car together, driving these same streets, thousands of times before. But on this day, pulling into our driveway felt different. My life, my mind, and my heart were fractured. There was no mending them until my family was together and well.

Joe helped me out of the car and up the front steps. Trying to start things off with a positive mindset, I called out, "I'm home!" as he opened the front door.

"Mommy!" Angelina shrieked when she saw me.

Every fiber of my being wanted to run to my daughter and swing her into my arms, but I was still sore from my C-section and winced with every step I took. As I padded toward her, I felt like I was walking in slow motion.

Fortunately, Angelina was happy to do the running for me. She sped toward me with open arms. "I missed you so much!" she said.

I beamed at her. She'd been seeing her daddy every day as he went back and forth from the hospital, but nothing was quite the same as a mother–daughter reunion. However, as happy as I was to see her, I couldn't shake the feeling that this was not how my return home after the birth of my twins was supposed to be. I should have been walking through the front door with Angelina's brother and sister nestled in my arms, ready to take our first photo at home as a family of five. Instead, the only things I held in my arms were a breast pump, my dirty clothes, and my medication. Worse, I didn't know if my babies would ever even make it home.

My mother was waiting for me. She had cleaned up the house, cooked for us, and done some laundry. No matter how much things had changed in my relationship with her as I'd grown up and become a mother myself, I would never outgrow my need for her, and she would always treat me like her baby girl.

"How are you feeling?" she asked, hugging me.

"I'm okay, Mom. I'm glad to be home, but I'm tired and need to lie down."

"Let me get you some water and help you to your room," she said.

I dragged myself up the short flight of stairs and down the hall. I paused in the doorway of Luke and Layla's nursery, taking in the empty room aside from two cribs, the rocker, and the changing table. I stepped inside and sat in the rocking chair, sighing as my body settled in.

My babies were tiny miracles. *They were still alive and, in my eyes, they were perfect, just like Angelina. They just need to grow and fully develop,* I told myself as I stared at the cribs. And I was finally home. But this room was empty when it should have been full. My thoughts were still just as chaotic as they had been during my time in the hospital. I felt as if I would never be able to relax. As I rocked back and forth, tears began streaming down my face and my sobs punctuated the silence. But only a few moments later, I heard Angelina's little footsteps coming up the stairs, Sky following behind her. I immediately silenced my cries and wiped my face. I couldn't let her see me upset. I had to keep myself together and stay strong for her sake.

Of course, astute as she was, she noticed right away that my eyes were red and swollen. "Mommy, what's wrong?" she asked.

"I'm just upset that your brother and sister can't be here with us. But hopefully they'll be home soon. They just need time to grow big and strong."

Angelina seemed satisfied with my response. After all, she was only five years old—too young to understand what being born at 26 weeks really meant. She gave me a big hug and then wandered back downstairs.

I stayed in the chair for a while longer, then pushed myself up and walked down the hallway into my room. The last time I had been in here, the sheets had been soaked with my blood and the bathroom had looked like the site of a massacre. Now, the bed was made with clean white sheets and the bathroom tile had been mopped until it gleamed. No one in the house would ever have guessed what had happened in these rooms less than one week prior.

While I was standing in the bathroom, I stood in front of the mirror, pulled my pants down a few inches, and examined my red, raised C-section incision, covered in stitches. It was far too raw, just like my emotions, for me to be able to envision what it would look like once it had healed, but the sight of the scar disoriented me. Just a week earlier, I had been worried about having a cesarean, and now it was already behind me— but not really.

I sighed and pulled my pants back up, then walked into my bedroom, turned down my comforter, and slipped into my bed. My pain medication and pure exhaustion quickly lulled me to sleep, but I kept jolting awake every hour or so. Having grown up in a peaceful, stable household, I didn't have any frame of reference to cope with all the turbulence I was experiencing. The last time I had slept in this bed, I had had my babies inside me. Now, Joe and I had to make some urgent decisions about how to give equal time to our kids. When I was at the hospital, I'd wonder, *How's Angelina doing? What am I making for dinner? Does she have gymnastics today?* And then as soon as I got home, I'd start wondering, *How are the twins doing? Are they okay?* And then there were the higher-level worries that kept me up at night: *How long will it take me to recover? How will I ever organize my life? Are Joe and I going to be able to afford all of this financially? Is the stress of our new life going to cause us to argue and tear us apart?* So many questions, so few concrete answers.

Joe and I tried to stagger our time at home, at the hospital, and eventually at work when I returned, so that each of us was always in a different place from the other. We were both exhausted, sleeping only a couple of hours at a time, but this was our new normal. We had a mission to give as much attention as we could to our two youngest children and to keep their older sibling as settled as possible, so we did what we had to do.

Although Joe and I were confident that the twins were receiving excellent care, I called the hospital compulsively to check on Luke and Layla when one of us couldn't be with them. "No news is good news," the nurses always assured me. "We will call you if there are any serious updates; otherwise, your babies will continue to undergo routine assessments and tests.

And remember that you can visit them anytime, day or night."

We took them at their word, believing that, just maybe, if we were with them as much as possible too, our presence would help them heal.

CHAPTER 12

The Baptismal Blessing

One of the biggest fears parents of micropreemies have is whether their children will actually survive. The thought that the twins might not make it another day was an ever-present reality.

"I want to baptize Luke and Layla, Joe. I'm worried. I'm very worried," I said to him as I paced the NICU one day when the twins were two weeks old. "I want them to have that blessing."

Joe and I were both raised in the Catholic faith. I had gone to church every Sunday as a child, and my mom was in constant, committed prayer—a practice that I had also adopted. In the Catholic tradition, baptizing a baby shortly after birth was a must. If something were to happen to the twins, we had to ensure that they would have the Lord's blessing and the gift of faith. In fact, it was extremely common for NICU babies to get baptized. The hospital staff even offered to provide a pastor, although we already had one in mind.

"I think we should have Father John come to the hospital to bless the babies. They deserve it, they need it, and I don't want any regrets," I told Joe.

We called upon the pastor who was part of our parish and knew our family well. When we told him about the babies, Father John said, "I heard. The whole congregation has been praying for you."

"Thank you," Joe and I mumbled simultaneously.

"How can I help?" Father John asked.

I spoke first. "Joe and I have been talking about it, and we've agreed that we'd like to get Luke and Layla baptized now while they are in the hospital. They need all the help they can get and this is important to us. We don't want to wait."

"Of course," Father John replied. "You tell me when, and I'll be there."

There was really nothing to prepare for—no beautiful dress or charming outfit, no gathering of family and friends, godparents and grandparents. Yet somehow it was still a beautiful morning and we made the best of it. We could only hope and pray that later on, one day we could give Luke and Layla a proper celebration for this important day.

Father John met us at the hospital. We welcomed him and escorted him back to the twins' room.

As he walked into the room, he was silent. We showed him to their incubators, lifting the blanket on each to give him a look.

"Wow, this is incredible. They're so tiny, yet such beautiful miracles," Father John said softly. "I've never witnessed anything like this before."

"Aren't they amazing?" I whispered as they slept.

Joe and I were used to seeing Luke and Layla by now, with all their tubes and wires and masks; they didn't look much different than they had the day they were born. But for Father John to be able to see past all their equipment to their natural radiance was something we hadn't expected.

When the ceremony began, Joe and I stood in prayer, heads down, in the middle of the room between Luke and Layla. Father John pulled his written prayers, a small chalice of holy water, and his notes from his briefcase. He had performed many baptisms in the past, but this one was unlike any other. His hands were shaking, but his voice was steady and his gentle words cleansed and re-energized our weary hearts.

After many prayers, we made our way to each baby's bedside. Father John wasn't sure how to administer the holy water, given their current state. I opened Layla's circular door and nodded at him. "Go ahead—it's okay to reach in."

Pushing back Layla's tiny hat, Father John poured a tiny droplet of blessed water on her forehead as he uttered many blessings. Joe and I stood silently. Immediately afterward, we walked over to Luke and did the same.

As Father John completed his final prayers and blessings, a sense of calmness and peace filled the air.

Luke and Layla did not have a single episode throughout the entire ceremony—no alarms going off, no nurses rushing in to nudge them to restart their breathing. They—and their parents—were at peace, at least for the time being.

february | *joe*

CHAPTER 13

Tag Teaming

A sappy movie was playing on the TV in the parents' break room. After spending six hours every evening in the NICU with Luke and Layla, surrounded by the sounds of monitors and medical personnel, I needed to break up the monotony and clear my head once in a while.

The room was quiet at 9:00 p.m., and none of the usual snacks seemed appealing, so I poured myself a cup of coffee and sat down in front of the television screen. Before I even realized it, tears were rolling down my cheeks. I just couldn't seem to find a happy medium—I was either hypersensitive or numb. After a few more minutes, I wiped my eyes, stood up, and headed back to my children.

As I walked down the halls, looking out the windows, I took in the raw energy of hospital life. Ambulance sirens screamed in the background. A helicopter slowly descended onto the roof. I never knew exactly what had just happened, or to whom, but I always knew it wasn't anything good. The fact that the hospital staff could tune out the suffering enough to do their jobs seemed like an impossibly heroic feat to me.

When I reached Luke and Layla's room, I plopped myself down on a chair in the corner. They slept peacefully while nurses came in and out, typing on computers, adjusting equipment, and responding to the babies' constant episodes. In the midst of the usual chaos, I sat still, thinking about how many aspects of our lives had changed so quickly.

About a month before the twins were born, I had chosen to go back to college to finish my bachelor's degree. This had been a goal of mine for years, and now I needed it more than ever. I thought about the conversation I'd had with Jenny months earlier.

"Now that we have twins coming, I need job security, and I don't feel as though I have that without a degree," I told her. "I need to do this—for me, for you, and for our kids."

Jenny nodded, maybe wondering how I was going to pull off this goal. She worked full-time at a real estate development company while pregnant with twins, and I had two jobs. How could we ever make time for school, especially once we had three kids? But I couldn't shake the idea that I had to do this.

Once the twins were born, I asked Jenny, "*Now* what should I do?" I was eager for any miraculous insight she might have about how I could ever pull off my plan. "I've started school several times, but there's always been something that kept me from finishing. I want this time to be different. Our kids will motivate me to keep going."

"Then do it. Finish. We'll figure it all out," Jenny said. "At this point in your life," she continued, "I don't think there's ever going to be a perfect time, and going to school will probably be even harder once the twins are home, so you might as well get started now."

I did as she said, but our routine immediately became a nonstop revolving door as a result—a series of tag-team efforts to balance our home and family life, our work lives, and now my school life. I spent my early morning and early evening hours with Angelina while Jenny was at work or at the hospital with Luke and Layla. I worked in the afternoons, we had dinner at home with Angelina, and after she went to bed I went to the hospital, often until midnight. I somehow found time on the weekends or in the middle of the night to complete the reading for my classes and write my required papers. Jenny and I were both running on minimal sleep and pure adrenaline.

No one ever could have guessed from Jenny's external demeanor—quiet, poised, and determined—that she was actually being crushed under the weight of her stress and fear about what the outcome for Luke and Layla might be. She was too stoic to lay her burdens upon anybody else. It was the way my wife had always been—strong and fierce. She prayed and hoped and let her faith take over. We both did. *This won't last forever,* I told myself. *We can take each difficult situation day by day.*

When things get tough, we get tougher. We had to. It was the only way we could get through this without crashing to the ground.

CHAPTER 14

New Normal

After the first few weeks, we had finally settled into a routine that seemed at least temporarily sustainable for all of us, as long as we refused to believe that sleep deprivation, lack of nourishment, constant worry, and a frantic pace of living would be our downfall. I had finally started to feel somewhat recovered while walking around, driving, and being able to stand on my own two feet again, but I was losing my baby weight too fast. After all, I never had time to eat because I was always on the run, and sometimes all the stress and anxiety nauseated me.

Every morning after I dropped off Angelina at school, I would drive straight to the hospital. My mother often met me there and spent a few hours with me while I tried to pump and participated in Luke and Layla's care. Most days, I would just sit in the green recliner in silence and stare at their beds, my mind racing. There was nothing I could do, nothing I could say, that would change my babies' current situation.

Joe and I were constantly on edge, but not with each other, fortunately. We knew we had to stick together; the only alternative was to fall apart. Angelina seemed to take our new normal in stride the best of all of us. She asked over and over, "When can I see my brother and sister?" but she was patient with our responses and she seemed to have a naturally optimistic outlook on the situation.

As the phone calls and text messages from well-wishers dwindled, aside from the select few who continued to check in, it was hard not to feel alone. Of course, it was understandable that people would not keep up the pace of their early outreach—they had to get back to their lives and didn't have unlimited time to worry about ours. I created an online journal through CaringBridge. It came recommended by my cousin in order to provide updates to our close friends and relatives. Not only did it allow me to reach out to more than 20 people at once, but I could also use it as a way to track Luke and Layla's progress and as an emotional release for myself. Just as drawing was a cathartic exercise for Angelina, I had always used journaling to work through my feelings. CaringBridge was a similar tool, and some of the people who might not otherwise have contacted us responded to Joe's and my posts with words of support that buoyed me: "My heart breaks for all of you. Stay strong; we love you and will continue to send prayers!" "These babies are not only miracles but warriors." "So glad things are trending in the right direction. Can't wait for them to come home."

Still, during the many days and nights when Joe and I sat quietly in the NICU, eyes glued to Luke and Layla's beeping, bubbling, blaring monitors, analyzing their heart rates and oxygen levels, dreading the next time they stopped breathing or their hearts arrested, wondering what would happen next, and knowing this ordeal was not ending anytime soon, we couldn't help but feel lonely and numb. Our lives were standing still while everyone else's kept moving. Some of the sounds from the endless hours in the NICU still trigger me now. Whenever I near a crosswalk, it emits a beeping "walk" signal that sounds exactly like one of the monitors my babies were hooked up to. I cringe every time I hear it.

Partly to give myself some sense of forward momentum and partly because I knew I couldn't jeopardize my job, which we needed now more than ever, I decided it was time for me to go back to work, even if only part-time. My employer had been supportive throughout this entire process, and I owed it to the company to start showing up. The parents' lounge at the hospital had a wonderful selection of snacks and drinks, all provided by the March of Dimes, an organization that supports parents of premature babies. It also had a desk with computers and telephones, where parents could sit and work as needed. I clearly wasn't the only parent who believed they needed to return to work. Because Luke and Layla spent most of the day sleeping while their bodies worked hard to grow,

Joe's and my jobs felt like a much-needed distraction.

Right under our noses, though, the twins were beginning to show signs of improvement. They had passed all of their critical exams so far, and their head scans were still clear—a huge milestone. After six days of intubation, Luke was extubated and finally given a SiPAP oxygen machine, similar to the one attached to Layla.

Despite their progress, the goings-on in the NICU were a constant reminder that our tenuous peace could be shattered at any moment—after all, the first few weeks of life are the most crucial. As I sat with the twins, listening to the white noise sounds from their oxygen machines, hearing the nurses chatting at their desk, and watching other mothers in their hospital gowns drifting down the hall, I felt for all of us. While each of our cases was different—some slightly better than ours, others worse—we were all unified in our daily challenge of facing the unexpected.

Some days, the sounds were nothing but horrific. I knew it was never good news when I heard sirens go off in rooms down the hall. It was as if the whole ward held its collective breath, every parent silently grateful that the flurry of nurses and doctors was passing their door, but also simultaneously praying for the family whose room they were rushing into.

One morning, peeking out from Luke and Layla's room, I noticed a congregation of nurses and doctors standing around a table full of medical equipment down the hall to my left. The look on their faces told me most of what I needed to know, but then I heard it—a wail so awful and unique that it was nearly indescribable: the cry of a mother whose baby had just died.

I was doubled over in my chair, feeling as if I might vomit, when a nurse walked in and broke my train of thought.

"The babies are going to get a feeding tube so we can begin to introduce breastmilk a few milliliters at a time," she said.

It took me a minute to focus on what she was saying; that other mother's cry was still echoing in my head. I wished so much that I could provide her with some sort of comfort. I found out later that they had had to perform emergency surgery on the baby down the hall who didn't make it. *That could easily have been Luke or Layla*, I kept thinking. But for now, they were alive, and I had to do my best to keep them that way.

Although I was still pumping as much as I could, donor milk was an invaluable supplement when I could not provide enough of my own milk for both babies. It never bothered me that they were drinking another mother's milk, as long as they were receiving the proper nutrients. I was so grateful for all the mothers who had donated their breastmilk. I hoped they knew it was being put to good use.

The nurse opened Luke's incubator and, with the help of another nurse, inserted an orange tube into his mouth, which needed to bypass his stomach and go into the small intestine. The feeding tube kept sliding up, as if it couldn't stay in the right position. Each time, the nurses had to push it back down his throat. One of them must have seen me cringing, because she said, "Don't worry; we do an X-ray to make sure the feeding tube is in the right spot. Because the babies are on high-pressure oxygen, they are not ready for the milk to go directly into their stomach as it might cause spit-ups, resulting in the babies having multiple episodes."

"Jeez, they get so many X-rays." I muttered, wondering if I should be worried about the high levels of radiation the twins were being exposed to so early in their lives.

"I know, but it's the only way we'll know the feeding tube is where it needs to be," the nurse said.

"It's a bit off," the other nurse said, as she reviewed the X-ray. They pulled the tube out and stuck it down Luke's throat again. Another X-ray. Another grimace from me. With each adjustment, I felt as if they were sliding the tube down my own throat. I could feel it scraping the back of my palate, and I gagged slightly. When Luke and Layla had been inside my body, I had been acutely aware that anything I ate, heard, or did would be experienced by my babies as well. Now it was happening in reverse.

"Still not right." The nurses stared at the most recent X-ray. "Try one more time," one said.

Luke began to squirm and writhe, and I had to look away, but I knew there was nothing I could do besides let the nurses do their job. Four tries later, they finally got the feeding tube secured in the right spot.

Luke's heart rate, oxygen levels, and blood count plummeted after that, and he had to undergo yet another transfusion. All I could do was place my finger in his tiny palm to try to comfort him. The nurses decided that because Luke was not tolerating his new SiPAP oxygen machine, the safest approach was to replace it with a NIPPV machine, which would put oxygen into his lungs more forcefully. It was very similar to being intubated, but without the breathing tube. Although it was what Luke needed for his numbers to normalize again, I couldn't help but think we were going backward, not forward.

The hospital staff had told Joe and me that visiting the NICU during the twins' care times, which occurred every three hours, would be valuable because I could be more hands-on in those intervals, helping to take the babies' temperature and change their diapers while they were somewhat awake. I wasn't allowed to hold them yet, so these basic activities were really my only chance to interact with them and give myself a modicum of normalcy.

"Would you like to change the babies' diapers?" the nurse asked me one day while I sat in my usual green recliner.

"Of course," I said, jumping right up while the nurse began unswaddling Layla, placing her on her back, and slowly waking her up from her peaceful sleep. I could tell my daughter was annoyed. Her little belly was puffed up like a balloon from all the excess air she was receiving from the oxygen. Sometimes, the swelling was so extreme that the nurses would attach an empty syringe to the feeding tube and manually suck the excess air out of the babies' abdomens. I could hear Layla squeal when the nurse "burped" her this way.

The nurse looked at me and said, "I know it can be scary sometimes, but don't worry—she's a strong girl, and you'll get used to handling her." She placed a diaper on Layla's bed. It was no more than three inches by three inches.

"Let me know if you need help," the nurse added, as I lifted Layla's pencil-thin legs, unwrapped her dirty diaper, and handed it to the nurse. I cleaned up Layla and attempted to put on the clean diaper, but maneuvering it all correctly took me a few tries because I moved so slowly, for fear of hurting her.

"Now we weigh the diaper," the nurse said. She turned away to weigh the diaper and then addressed me again, handing me a thermometer. "Just lift her arm and place it gently in her armpit."

I lifted Layla's arm, placed the thermometer under her armpit, and waited a few seconds until it beeped. I caressed her cheek while I waited. "Great—her temperature is normal," the nurse said. She then swapped out Layla's nose prongs for a more delicate mask that went over her nose for her oxygen. The prongs were very irritable, so putting the mask on instead made Layla more comfortable.

I gingerly embraced my daughter as best I could. I gave her a hand hug. I wrapped my gloved fingers around her head and fragile feet. Longing pulsed through my heart as I let go and allowed the nurses to complete their assessments.

The next day, I watched the babies sleep for hours. For a practical, get-'er-done personality like mine, the uneventful days were almost as difficult as the hectic ones. Pumping breastmilk was getting old, and the hours dragged by more slowly than I'd ever experienced. To pass the time, I dipped into my nostalgic memory banks, remembering my early twenties, when I spent most every weekend going out with my friends, dancing the night away, eating good food, and having fun—not a care in the world. *Not in a million years would I ever have expected then that I would end up where I am right now, I thought.*

A hospital administrator walked in and winked when she saw me pacing. "Hi, Mama. How about some paperwork to keep you busy?" She handed me a stack of papers to review. "You can hand these to the nurse once you've completed them."

Filling out forms was the last thing I wanted to do. In an attempt to postpone the inevitable, I scanned the room until my eyes settled on a bag attached to a mask hanging above Layla's bed.

"What's that bag for?" I asked.

"It's a bag-mask that pumps oxygen through a bag delivering 100% oxygen in order to resuscitate the baby in case they stop breathing and don't respond to us," the nurse said. "It's basically CPR, but since an adult's mouth is far too big to give CPR to a preemie, this is what we use."

Just looking at it nauseated me. *How much can one family handle?* I wondered, wincing again.

CHAPTER 15

Valentine's Day

On Valentine's Day morning, Joe and I left a bag full of candy, a teddy bear, and a balloon on the kitchen counter for Angelina.

"Thank you, Mommy and Daddy!" she squealed as she came down the stairs and saw her gifts.

"Happy Valentine's Day, honey!" I said. "I made you some cupcakes to take to school to enjoy with your friends, and we'll have a nice dinner later together when you get home."

"I made something for Luke and Layla!" she said. She walked over to her craft table, pulled out her drawing pad, and grabbed two pictures she had drawn for them. I felt my eyes widen as I examined them, noticing that on each page she had written their name and drawn underneath a baby wearing a cape and flying high in the sky, with the inscription "Superhero."

"They're fighters, Mommy," Angelina said while I continued to gape at her work. "They're strong and brave and are my superheroes. Can you hang these in their hospital room?"

My eyes filled with tears as I said, "Honey, this is so sweet—your brother and sister are going to love these." I bent down to give her a long, tight hug.

Angelina smiled, then grabbed her teddy bear, ate a piece of chocolate, and went back upstairs to finish getting ready for school. Her innocence was bliss. I knew that drawing was a coping mechanism for her, but she never showed any distress. *How can a five-year-old be so thoughtful and understanding during a time like this?* I marveled. *I might never know, but what a blessing.*

After I dropped off Angelina at school, I headed to the hospital. I couldn't bring anything into the NICU aside from a card from me and the pictures that Angelina had drawn for her siblings. To prevent germs, the pictures had to be laminated before they could be hung in their room. "Your sister brought you a Valentine's Day gift," I said out loud to the twins while I hung the drawings on either side of the room. As I stared at the photos, I quickly noticed a new sound in the background coming from Layla's oxygen machine. It was a constant bubble noise that almost sounded like you were in a spa.

I began to walk over to her oxygen machine when the doctor walked in to give me an update. "Is Layla on a different type of oxygen support?" I asked.

"Yes. It's a good sign! She has been switched to a bubble CPAP machine, which is a step down from the SiPAP. She is now receiving one constant pressure, which is gentler and better for the lungs, instead of forced mechanical air. Luke will eventually get there too."

I took a sigh of relief. I was happy that she was moving forward, but also nervous at the fact that she was now receiving less respiratory help.

"Also, starting next week and every Tuesday thereafter," the doctor continued, "the ophthalmologist will come by to give the babies their eye exams. They'll be looking for anything abnormal, specifically something called retinopathy of prematurity. We want to ensure the blood vessels are growing as they should be. Typically, this is an exam we advise parents not to watch. It's not painful, but it is very uncomfortable and a bit disturbing to witness."

"Also, the babies have been tolerating breastmilk really well," the nurse said, turning toward me again. "So well, in fact, that I removed the PICC line that administers their TPN because they no longer need the extra fluids. They barely spit up now, so we've increased their intake in the hopes that we can feed them more and they in turn will receive more nutrients to grow."

I wanted all the tubes and needles to come out, but the fact that even one of the many devices attached to them was finally coming off was a victory in itself. I thought back to the early days after the twins' birth, when one of my first interactions with them was giving them colostrum on a Q-tip. As I placed the precious drops on their lips, they slowly slurped up the liquid, eyes closed. *And look at them now*, I thought, *doing it on their own*. I reminded myself never to lose sight of my gratitude for moments like this.

"Another IV line out means their chances of infection will drop dramatically. And you know what else it means, right?" The nurse winked.

I didn't dare let myself think it, but the doctor was still smiling and nodding. "It's safe to hold Luke, if you'd like," she said.

"Yes, of course!" I said, but I couldn't help but add, "Are you sure it's okay?"

"I don't think Layla is quite ready yet; her heart rate has been dropping off and on quite a bit recently, and I don't want to further stress her system by removing her from her incubator, but I think Luke is ready for some skin-to-skin contact with Mom. Pull up a chair and put on this hospital gown."

I started to tremble. It had been two and a half weeks since Luke had heard my heartbeat, smelled my skin, and felt the tenderness of my embrace. After four months together with him in my womb, I had missed him desperately these last weeks. Now, it was finally time to reunite.

It took two nurses to get him out safely and into my arms. One nurse reached in, unswaddled him, and lifted him out while another nurse maneuvered his oxygen tubes and leads. He was finally off the NIPPV machine and back on the SiPAP, which looked like a crinkled vacuum hose as it extended toward me. The three different wires attached to his chest to monitor his heart hung from him like a spiderweb. His feeding tube was still in place, and the pulse oximeter on his tiny foot emitted a red light.

The nurse moved Luke slowly so that nothing came out of place. I sat anxiously awaiting him in the chair at his bedside. When she placed him on my chest, I began to cry quietly as I pressed his skin against mine. The nurses had no problem handling two-pound babies with finesse. I wasn't nearly as sure that I could do the same.

A second later, however, I forgot what I had ever been afraid of. *This is natural; this is right; this is exactly what I've been needing*, I thought, as I gazed down at the soft fuzz on Luke's delicate back. Finally, we could partake in the miracle that should have happened seconds after their birth.

Luke was so minute that I could fit him in my left hand while I cupped his legs and bottom into my palm. His head sat sideways over my heart as it beat into his ear. I could feel his chest heaving in and out as his own pulse raced. I bent down to kiss his head softly over and over.

The nurse slipped out of the room as my son and I both got lost in the moment. I rocked him and sang him a lullaby while he nestled under my hospital gown. It was perfect—almost. As with all of my recent parenting experiences, I was torn between two worlds. I looked over at Layla, alone, enclosed, and I knew I wouldn't feel complete until she, too, was snuggled against my chest, right next to her brother.

I also wished that Joe or Angelina could have been there with me to witness such a special moment. It almost felt wrong, holding him without having them nearby, but I would share every detail with them when I saw them later.

While I continued to rock Luke, I remembered a story my mother had told me about her brother and sister, who had been born more than 50 years earlier in a small village in Portugal. "You know," my mom had said, "my siblings and I were all born at home with a midwife. Things weren't as promising as they are today. Your uncle was a twin, and born very small. His temperature would not stabilize; he was cold and very weak. He survived only because your grandfather would sit by the fire, hold him tightly on his chest, and cover him with blankets to keep him warm. Your grandmother would squeeze breastmilk into his mouth because my brother didn't have the strength to suck the milk. Back then, we didn't have the same kinds of hospitals, wonderful nurses, or machines to keep us stable. It was survival of the fittest, and, unfortunately, my brother's twin sister didn't survive."

Even at the time, I hadn't been able to imagine what my grandmother had endured. Now more than ever, I knew she was right—about all the help surrounding me, and about how privileged I was to experience this precious moment.

Suddenly, Luke became restless and his monitors began to beep, alerting the nurses that he needed attention. I knew they needed to put him back, but as they rushed in to swaddle him and place him on his belly in his bed, all I could think was, *Just like that, he's been taken from me again.*

A few days later, the nurses informed me that I could hold Layla. This time, I made sure Joe could be there so that he didn't have to miss out.

It was very rare that Joe and I got to be at the hospital together. Knowing that, the nurses were prepared for our arrival. As we entered the twins' room and approached them, I noticed the nurse was buttoning up the bottom of a white onesie. Luke and Layla both finally had clothes on. Their arms and legs swam inside the cloth because they were still so small that even preemie clothes didn't fit yet.

The nurse smiled and said, "Your babies are getting so big! Now that they've reached 2.5 pounds, we can switch them from a skin control environment to an air-controlled environment, meaning that the incubator is one constant temperature and they have to learn to maintain their own body temperature. Don't worry, we'll still keep them swaddled up nice and warm, but you can start bringing in preemie clothes for them to wear. Just make sure you wash them beforehand."

"Absolutely!" I said, beaming at her. I had onesies piled up at home and had just been waiting, hoping, wondering if one day the twins would get to wear them. Now, I could finally provide them with their own clothing. The little things were what hit home the most.

"Oh, and once they grow to 3.5 pounds, they will graduate to an open crib!" the nurse continued as she finished swaddling Layla.

We noticed that our recliners had been pushed close to each other in the center of the room. Hospital gowns for both Joe and me hung on the chairs. Two nurses stood ready to transfer each baby to us. We put on our gowns and sat down while they positioned Luke on Joe's chest and Layla on mine. Their breathing tubes extended from their faces, around our bodies, and into the machines.

As Joe and I embraced our children, a tender silence engulfed us. The low lights, the rhythm of the machines, and the sound of the oxygen tanks became hypnotic. I teared up again as I watched Joe gazing at his firstborn son. I could only imagine what he was thinking.

I asked one of the nurses to capture this moment of the four of us together. It was the picture that should have been taken the day Luke and Layla were born. Angelina was the missing piece of the puzzle, but I hoped that we would have a photo of our entire family of five soon.

When I heard one of the monitors start to beep and noticed bright lights coming from Layla's side of the room, Joe and I both looked up at the flashing numbers.

Layla began to squirm and fuss on my chest, so I lifted her gently and nudged her arm, imitating what the nurses did to get her to breathe. "Come on, baby girl," I said. Slowly, the numbers began to climb back up and the beeping stopped.

The nurse didn't even have to step in; she simply watched in awe.

"You're learning, I see," she said, smiling.

I grinned back at her and said, "I guess my maternal instincts kicked in. It scares me every time, but at least I understand what's happening now."

As I stared at my daughter's beautiful face, closed eyes, and delicate, fair skin, she grinned softly at me. I couldn't help but smile back while simultaneously brushing away a tear of joy. I felt my heart miss a beat, but I welcomed it because I knew, even if only for a moment, that my babies were okay.

CHAPTER 16

Please Breathe

One day after work, I went to the NICU to meet my mom. She usually greeted me with a warm smile, but on this particular afternoon, I caught her eyes scanning my body. "You look so thin," my mom said. "That's not a good thing when you're breastfeeding. You need to eat." She used her softest, most maternal tone, and I knew she was right.

I had always been thin, but I had lost all my baby weight almost immediately after the twins were born, and now I weighed even less than I had before I got pregnant. I was living mostly on chips, protein bars, and bottled water from the parents' lounge at the hospital.

"Sitting down to eat is honestly the last thing on my mind right now," I told my mother. "The stress and constant running around don't help either. But don't worry, Mom. I'll be fine," I said, as much to convince myself as to reassure her.

I continued, "You know I couldn't get through this without you and Dad. Thank you for being with me. I don't feel as lonely when you're here."

Suddenly, an alarm began to wail. As much as I was used to the sound by now, my whole body tensed every time it started up. And when I looked over at the flashing lights coming from Layla's monitor, I knew something was different this time.

Mom and I stared at the monitor. The line that indicated Layla's heartbeat had suddenly plunged all the way to the bottom. Her heart rate read 0—meaning her heart wasn't even beating—and her oxygen levels plummeted from 98 percent to 5 percent. Meanwhile, my own heart began to race.

The sound of footsteps filled the hall, and six nurses rushed into the room. I recognized nurses from other departments of the NICU and flashbacks of what I had witnessed weeks earlier played back in my head. The sound of that poor mother's cries had never left me.

The nurses didn't waste any time opening the top of Layla's incubator. One nurse unwrapped her. Another tugged on her tiny arm and massaged her leg. Yet another grabbed her like a rag doll, rubbing her and patting her back, saying, "Come on, Layla, breathe."

My mother and I had risen out of our recliners and stood by helplessly. I honestly thought I might go into cardiac arrest when I realized that Layla wasn't responding to any of the nurses' attempts to revitalize her. An ashen blue color was slowly taking over her tiny body.

"Bag!" I heard a nurse shout.

I gasped as another nurse grabbed the bag-mask—formally called an AMBU bag—off the wall to administer CPR. It had a mask on one end, a middle piece that looked like a grenade, and something that resembled a crumpled plastic bag on the other end. I had been terrified of this apparatus ever since the first time I had seen it hanging over the twins bedside, and now it was being used on my daughter in front of my own eyes. The mask went over her face. Nurses rhythmically squeezed the big red pump, counting the repetitions as they forced air into Layla's lungs.

This can't be happening, I thought, feeling my eyes prick with tears. This was the moment I had hoped and prayed and willed not to happen during all of these boring days. "Come on, Layla! Come on, baby girl!" one nurse shouted.

I was standing in the middle of the room. I became vaguely aware of my mother's presence beside me and glanced over at her. Her lips moved in silent prayer as she looked away.

I was praying too, willing Layla to be strong. *Please breathe. Please breathe. Please breathe. Please come back to us.*

Too many medical personnel were crowding around Layla for me to have a clear view of her. I knew her brother was sleeping peacefully across the room, but I couldn't see him well either. I could only hear the nurses' desperate calls and the sounds of monitors going awry.

The nurses were counting the compressions they were administering to her fragile chest.

"Breathe." They pumped the air into her mouth.

"Compressions. One, two, three, breathe…"

I thought of Joe and Angelina. What would I say to them?

Suddenly, it sounded like the machines were staggering to right themselves. I saw Layla's heartbeat and the line indicating her breathing leap across the screen. I held my breath.

"She's back," a nurse finally said. Pink started creeping back across Layla's head, chest, and back. I had no idea how much time had elapsed. All I knew was that I wasn't even close to being able to calm down—I had too much adrenaline surging through my veins. *What was that, and why did it even happen? How long was Layla out? Was it long enough to cause damage from lack of oxygen? Is she regressing?* My thoughts came almost too quickly for me to hear them in my own head. I knew these kinds of incidents happen more often with preemies, but, given that we were already a month or two in, I must have allowed myself to become just a hair less vigilant—to relax, however briefly or unconsciously, into a sense that my daughter was going to be one of the lucky ones. *How naive I was*, I realized now. *Things really can go wrong at any moment. We're not even close to being out of the woods.*

My tears came in a flood as I lowered myself into the recliner next to my mother. She rubbed my back while I sobbed. The nurses cleaned up the room and filtered out, leaving us alone with the twins. I sat until my heart rate had finally slowed enough for me to dial Joe.

"It was terrifying," I said, after I told him the news. "Absolutely terrifying. I'm still so scared. Out of nowhere! Layla was totally fine one second and not the next! The nurses were so amazing—I watched as they saved her life. I can't believe I just witnessed that and couldn't do anything to help."

Joe was speechless at first. "My poor girl." He spoke as his voice cracked. "I can't believe that happened to her and, on top of that, you had to witness it," Joe said. "But look, she's okay now and I'm sure they are going to keep an even closer eye on her now. Let's try to stay focused and keep moving forward."

Focusing was the last thing I could do at that moment, but I knew he was only trying to keep me calm and to mitigate his own worry.

As I hung up the phone, I looked over at my mother. "I don't know if he completely understands what we just went through," I said to her. "I don't think anyone could possibly understand what that was like unless they witnessed it with their own eyes." But I was also certain that Joe was on his knees in that moment, thanking God that our younger daughter was still alive.

For the next few days, I didn't want to leave my babies' side.

"I can't stay away from the NICU, not after that," I told my mom. "What if it happens again? What if it happens at night when Joe and I are both asleep at home? Or what if I'm at my office? I'll never be able to forgive myself."

"We'll figure it out. I'll sit with them when you're at work," my mom assured me. But when I looked into her eyes, I noticed that they were filled with tears. I could only imagine how many memories of my brother and sister, both gone too soon, were coming up for her. I tried to find some comfort in that by telling myself that they were Luke and Layla's guardian angels and had been with us all along. But on top of that, I also sensed how terrified my mom must be after having almost lost Layla and now realizing that she could lose Luke at any moment as well.

Saying goodbye and walking out each day without knowing what the next few hours would bring before I returned was the hardest thing to do. As I drove nervously to work that afternoon, I couldn't get my mind around the fact that I was supposed to walk into an office after what had just happened and act composed around my colleagues. The incident with Layla filled every crevice of my brain.

It took me a long time to recover emotionally from that episode. Just when I was thinking their conditions were trending in the right direction, this surprise had come up. At first, I spent most of my time wondering, *Is this going to happen again? Will it all get worse from here? Am I going to get a phone call in the middle of the night with bad news? I'm not sure I can handle this much longer.* But as Joe and I talked, prayed, continued to trust the NICU team, and spent time with all three of our children, I slowly began to trust that life would somehow return to normal.

CHAPTER 17

Dinner with Daddy

It was a Saturday morning. The cadaver lay lifeless on the table. I watched the surgeon sear through the skin with a bovie. The smell of burned flesh filled the air in the bio-skills lab where we were helping to train the surgeon in a complex procedure utilizing the products that our company manufactured and sold. The scrub technicians looked to me for guidance on what instrument to employ next. After all, these were my company's products they were using.

I was an expert at helping surgeons learn the specifics of foot and ankle surgeries. Building relationships, support- ing surgeons, and selling orthopedic screws, plates, and other implants to surgeons was what I did best. Like my parents coming to America, I had started from scratch, built my terri- tory, developed a solid client base, and hit my quota each time.

Despite my commitment and growth, corporate leadership was hard to please. I had asked them for a raise in November, when I knew the twins were coming. I had said, "Listen, I've been here for a long time, and I know I'm underpaid. If I were to go somewhere else, my base salary and total compensation package would be much higher."

"Well, Joe," leadership said, "We don't have the budget to give you a raise. And you can't go anywhere else for at least a year because you have a noncompete clause in your contract with us, which we will not hesitate to enforce!" If I knew then what I know now, it would all have made more sense. The company was positioning themselves to sell to a giant competitor.

The tension between us only worsened from there. A few weeks after Luke and Layla were born, leadership called and said, "Your numbers are dropping. You're not out there selling as much as you should be."

"I know. Everything that's been going on with my kids and trying to keep my family together has been draining, both mentally and physically," I said.

I knew what they were saying was true, but after all I'd done for the company for over a decade, I thought they would have been more understanding about the extraordinary situation I was now navigating. Instead, they said, "We need you growing numbers. You have a job to do. You have to set aside your personal crisis and go out and do your job."

I had long suspected that they were threatened by the success and the relationships my colleague and I had achieved over the past decade, but this conversation solidified my understanding that they didn't care at all about me or my family. *All they cared about were the sales numbers, I realized. It doesn't even matter to them that my situation is only temporary—they are never going to cut me any slack.*

I couldn't hold back anymore. "You never even ask how I'm doing, how my kids are doing. They're in the frickin' hospital!" I screamed.

"It's a sensitive situation," leadership replied, without a trace of empathy or elaboration.

I had already been considering branching out on my own in July, two months after the twins' due date. My area of sales expertise, total ankle replacements and complex rear foot deformities, not to mention my decade-long relationships with all the surgeons and hospital staff, was a rarity in my territory. I was attending almost all of the complex surgeries in Washington, D.C., and Virginia for my team. For this reason, the heads of another company had already been courting me to join them, but I was skeptical. It was a small company with an elementary product line that was in its infancy. They wanted me to help them navigate this new territory and help them grow a sales team and introductions to key opinion leaders who could come in and redesign and improve the products.

However, I had been forced to put that idea on hold after Luke and Layla's early arrival. Now, however, amid this increasing tension with the leadership team and my new knowledge that I would never be appropriately compensated for my work, I knew I should trust my gut and go for it. I decided then that I would give my existing local sales team and surgeons the respect they deserved and transition things correctly versus quitting from one day to another. I went to a colleague I trusted and who had been shadowing me and said, "I don't know that I'm going to be able to do this much longer. I need you to double down on applying yourself and learning. I want to teach you everything you need to know about total ankle replacements in the next 30 days."

"Are you going to leave?" she asked.

I said no—I told her I was just going to take some time off, to avoid causing any panic or disrupting the team—but in the back of my mind I knew my time at the company was over. I wanted to teach her how to support the doctors through surgery on her own so that I could move on knowing the surgeons would be left in good hands. It was a tough decision for me, given I enjoyed working with my local sales team, but I was doing what I felt was right for my family.

When talking with Jenny about the situation, I said, "I've worked so hard for this company for over 10 years now, but I'm just a number. I have done my time, I've built my relationships, and it's time to move on and start my own business for us."

"Of course," Jenny said. "Do what you need to do." She always had my back. Either she supported my decisions outright or we talked through a challenge until we arrived at the solution that would be best for our family.

"Our family is what's most important," I said. "No fear is going to take that away from me." Having grown up in a family where pressure, anxiety, and fear had gotten the better of my parents, I would not let that happen to us.

Thirty days later, I put in my resignation letter.

My brief sense of triumph quickly gave way to questions: *Am I ready for the next step? Do I actually have what it takes to start my own medical device distributorship? Can I build a team from scratch?* Although I had begun the process of finishing my college degree and knew that I would achieve my goal this time, I also knew I wouldn't feel fully credible until I had my diploma in hand.

I had always known that I was good with people, but I hadn't gotten good grades in college when I was there originally because I never applied myself. *Maybe I'm just street smart*, I thought. *Maybe I'm just charismatic and good at selling people stuff. Maybe I'm just not book smart.* I had never been put in a scenario that really challenged my intelligence. But once I went back to school this time, it felt like an insurance policy for my family. Every time I looked at my children, I thought, *I have to get this piece of paper. I have to get it so that I can get a future leadership position if needed. And I don't want my own kids ever telling me they don't need to go to college because I didn't.*

As committed as I was to graduating, one night I decided to put my schoolwork aside. I had been so focused on work, school, and Luke and Layla that I needed a moment to breathe.

I found Angelina in her room, knelt down in front of her, looked into her soft, gleaming eyes, and said, "Honey, I think we need a daddy–daughter date. Mommy's at the hospital with the twins. Would you like to go out to eat with me tonight?"

"Yes, Daddy!" Angelina bounced a little on her toes.

"Where would you like to go?"

"I want to get my favorite cheese raviolis down the street!"

I smiled. "You got it. Anything for my girl."

While I drove us to our family's favorite Italian restaurant, I glanced in the rearview mirror at the little girl in the backseat. For the first five years of her life, she had been my world. I wanted to have a moment with her, just the two of us, the way things had been before the twins were born and everything changed overnight. We both needed a reset.

Even though Angelina worked hard to keep it together, I could tell she was confused. She was always wise beyond her years. She asked a lot of questions about her brother and sister. Why couldn't she see them? Why were they in the hospital when everyone else's baby siblings got to come home? Why were her mom and I there so much?

As the victim of an unstable childhood, I had promised myself I would try to learn from the mistakes I saw with my own eyes growing up and to raise my children in a different way, as much as I could manage it. It was essential to me that Angelina knew I was always available to her and that she could come talk to me about anything. Jenny and I never wanted her to feel shafted or worry that she wasn't just as important to us as her brother and sister. And that was what I was trying to do by taking her to dinner.

The restaurant was just down the street, and we were seated minutes later. Angelina loved our waiter, who always welcomed us like old friends.

We relaxed into the warm, quiet atmosphere and dug into plates of steaming ravioli. Angelina glowed while she ate. Her long, dark hair framed her green eyes and gentle face. In between bites, she rewarded me with big smiles. Every moment I spent with her was worth it, and believing in myself was the right choice.

"I know Mommy and Daddy have been very busy lately with your brother and sister," I said, as Tony brought us gelato. "Our family is going through a lot of changes, but hopefully it will all be over soon. It's very hard for all of us, especially Mommy. I want you to know that this is not forever. Eventually, your brother and sister will come home and our life will go back to normal. And at least you get to spend more time with Vovó now!"

"I know, Daddy," Angelina said. "I know Luke and Layla just need to grow and get better. I just can't wait to meet them. Now, let's have some gelato! Dig in!"

How is this child so wise beyond her years? I wondered, picking up my spoon. But I also knew that having two parents who were as committed to each other as they were to their kids had given her the best foundation possible. Jenny and I always made sure to focus on our marriage, despite our many fears. We were both practical, determined, focused, and utterly devoted to teamwork. We didn't see each other much those days, and when we did, we talked mostly about logistics or the trauma we were experiencing. But I hoped that one day soon, we would all be together under the same roof as a family of five. That visual seemed like nothing short of a miracle, but anything was possible.

CHAPTER 18

Longing

Joe wasn't the only one who worried about Angelina and wanted to make sure he spent one-on-one time with her. We never wanted her to feel unwanted or pushed to the side—she had every right to get as much attention as her brother and sister were getting from us.

Joe and I did our best to keep her life as stable and normal as possible. She continued to participate in sports, have playdates, go to school, and spend time with us in the evenings before bed. She and I loved going out for frozen yogurt and drawing pictures together. I drove her to all her gymnastics and dance classes so we could talk on the way.

We also kept a calendar at home for the twins. Angelina and I crossed off each day leading up to their due date, the day we expected them to come home. Eventually, we also started noting their increasing weight and any other milestones worth tracking. By March, they had each gained a pound, which was a huge deal. It helped Angelina to understand that her brother and sister were growing and getting stronger every day—and it was a good reminder for me, too.

When Angelina got quiet, I could usually tell she had a lot on her mind. She was like me that way.

"Honey, what's the matter?" I asked during one of our frozen yogurt dates.

"Nothing. I'm okay," she said.

I knew I had to dig deeper. "Are you sure? Is it the twins? Are you upset that Mom and Dad aren't around as much?"

"It's just... I'm worried about Luke and Layla. And you're always at the hospital. I miss you," she said, hanging her head.

"Angelina, you know how much we love you. Nothing will ever change that. But you also need to understand that now you have a brother and sister whom we also love just as much. Promise me that if you ever feel sad, you'll come talk to me or Dad?"

"I know, I will," she said, passively stirring her now-melting frozen yogurt with her plastic spoon. "I just don't understand why I can't go visit them. I'm their sister. And why do they have to wear a mask and have tubes in their mouth, like I see in the pictures?" she asked.

I felt terrible that she had to see her siblings with scary medical equipment attached to them, but it was either that or not share photos of the twins with her at all. Joe and I thought it was better that Luke and Layla were nearly as real to Angelina as they were to us, but now I realized how confusing our approach must have been. "Those masks and tubes help them breathe and eat because they're not strong enough to do it on their own yet. But don't worry. Soon enough you'll be able to visit them—I promise."

I just want Luke and Layla home now," Angelina said.

"Me too, honey. Me too," I told her, squeezing her little hand across the table.

That night, Angelina sat in her room with Sky, who never left her side. She began to pet her, play tug-a-war with a chew toy and then gave her a big hug before she sat down at the desk in her room to draw. Not only was Angelina good at drawing, but I knew, just like being with Sky, drawing was also a way for her to cope with what was going on in her life. If drawing helped her get through it, I was all for it.

She grabbed her notepad and picked up her pencil. She drew the sky first, a pretty blue, and then green grass along the bottom. She slowly added our family, all five of us. Together. It was perfect.

late march | jenny

CHAPTER 19

Regret

———

By now, we had gotten used to not having nearly as many friends and relatives check on us or stop by to drop off food and gifts. After all, everyone had their own lives to deal with, so they had mostly resorted to waiting for updates from us on CaringBridge.

"I think people are just scared to get in the way," Joe assured me. "They probably have good intentions, but they're not sure what to say."

"I understand that people don't know what to do or what to say," I agreed. "But these are the times when you realize who is closest to you and who shows up when you need them the most. I'm only going through one of the hardest times of my life."

"I know. I hear you. Don't let it bother you. We have enough to worry about right now," Joe said.

After this exchange, we sat quietly for a few minutes. Joe and I had never felt as if we needed to fill every moment with conversation to feel close to each other. And in those stressful days, silence often seemed like the most natural emotional response, both at home and around other people. Most of the time, I didn't feel up to having awkward conversations about my kids.

On the rare occasion that I did get together with friends, they would smile at me and say, "Everything's going to be okay. The babies will make it through, and so will you."

I knew they were doing their best to comfort me, but I always found myself fighting back tears, wondering, *How can they have any clue about what I'm feeling? They have no concept of the magnitude of my stress and trauma. And if I can't even talk to my friends about what I'm going through without crying, then it's definitely not worth seeing people who don't know me as well.* But I had to tell myself that it wasn't their fault and that the ones who did try were doing their best to comfort me.

I finally decided to tear myself away from the hospital to attend a family event with Joe. I knew that the room would be filled with acquaintances and members of our extended family, and that I would likely face a barrage of questions, but I hadn't seen anyone besides my immediate family for a long time. My world had shrunk to a minuscule size as I became laser-focused on my family's survival. *Maybe,* I thought, *this will be good for us.*

But I knew I had made a mistake as soon as I arrived and people flocked around me, asking, "How are you feeling? How are the babies?"

I knew what they wanted to hear, so I said, "We're doing okay," but as soon as I spoke the words, my eyes filled with tears and I instantly thought, *I shouldn't have come. This was a bad idea. I shouldn't have sacrificed time with my kids to be here.*

After too many of these interactions, I retreated to the corner where my parents and my brothers were sitting and mostly avoided people for the rest of the celebration. Joe was more social, mingling with the other guests and most likely putting on a brave face, but I was too drained and too guilt-ridden for that.

How can I say, "My babies are okay, and I'm okay," when I'm really not? I screamed inside. *I just want to go home.*

CHAPTER 20

One Step Forward, Three Steps Back

The days were beginning to blur together, yet things were looking up. Even though we still had a long way to go, Luke and Layla were growing steadily and getting stronger and stronger every day. They continued to gain weight, their feedings were increasing, and their need for additional oxygen began to dwindle. The first week of April, they were removed from their CPAP oxygen machines. The uncomfortable masks and nose prongs they had worn for months were no more. Now, only a small, thin plastic tube known as a cannula was placed under their nostrils and taped to their faces. They were on the lowest-pressure oxygen machine and working their way off it completely. That was a terrifying process, given all they had been through—especially Layla, who had had the most trouble breathing on her own. But if the doctors believed my babies were ready for the next phase, I trusted them. Unless Joe and I had to make a decision about something major, they chose and executed the steps that they deemed necessary for each baby. If the twins needed X-rays, they got X-rays, whether Joe and I were there or not. If they needed a blood transfusion, they got a blood transfusion. The doctors acted as specific needs arose, the nurses followed up on whatever instructions they received, and everyone kept Joe and me updated on a need-to-know basis.

One evening in mid-April, the doctor told me that I could attempt to bottle-feed Luke and Layla to see how they would do. Premature infants can have a hard time understanding the concept of sucking and breathing simultaneously, but it was time to try.

When I arrived at the NICU the next morning, the nurses were assessing Luke and Layla when I noticed that the enclosed incubators that had been the twins' beds for months were gone. I looked all around the room to make sure I was in the right place, before I noticed that both babies had been relocated to their very own open cribs, right at room temperature. The sight of them after they had achieved this milestone felt like the greatest victory yet. I didn't even care that I hadn't been present for the crib transfer; I was just so grateful and happy that it had happened at all. As long as a change was positive, that was all I could ask for.

I moved on to my next pressing question: "So, can I still try to bottle-feed today?" I asked.

"Of course. You're just in time for their next feeding. I'll grab their bottles and some of your breastmilk, and let's give it a go."

While I waited for the nurse to return, I reached into each crib and stroked my babies' cheeks, which were finally exposed to the air. Still, I knew their struggles were far from over. They both still needed to learn how to bottle-feed and breathe at the same time so that they could get off their feeding tubes and begin growing more rapidly.

"Here you go, Mom." The nurse was back. She handed me a bottle the size of my finger. It held only a few milliliters of milk.

She propped Layla up on her bottom, placing one hand behind her neck to hold her upright.

"Go ahead and see if she latches on."

I gently placed the bottle in Layla's mouth, and she grabbed it immediately with her birdlike lips, as if she had been waiting for it all along. She began sucking so fast that she forgot to breathe, and a round of alarms sounded in the room. I quickly released the bottle, letting her catch her breath.

"It's okay," the nurse said. "This is totally normal. She still needs to figure out how to take it more slowly and find her rhythm."

These bottle-feeding lessons continued throughout the afternoon. Luke had a much harder time grasping the concept, but I knew he would catch on eventually. Each day, they were introduced to a larger quantity of breastmilk to train their stomachs to tolerate more and more. Their feeding tubes were now in their noses, not their mouths, so they could both bottle-feed and breastfeed. The nurses also gave them pacifiers while they slept, to further help with their coordination. The more milk they were able to drink out of the bottle, the less they were given through their feeding tubes. Once they were drinking the full four ounces of milk on schedule without sounding the alarms, their feeding tubes would be removed. Each moment I was able to both breastfeed and bottle-feed my babies was a monument to our success.

Luke and Layla were also officially relocated from their original room called the Rainforest, to a beautiful corner room called the River, an area of the NICU that was considered intermediate care. Their new home had windows everywhere, which sent sunbeams dancing through the space and over the twins' cribs; the contrast with the Rainforest, which was always dark and felt like a bunker, was equivalent to the difference between a roadside motel and an upscale boutique hotel.

I continued to visit the NICU every day. I had stood by, watching the nurses tend to Luke and Layla, for so long that I was ready to step in. Each of my visits had more and more of a purpose now that I could pick the twins up when I wanted to, change their clothes, complete their assessments by myself, sponge-bathe them, and put them to sleep. That was my favorite part—sitting peacefully with them in the rocking chair in their room and singing to them as they drifted off. Their facial features were starting to become more distinct, and I couldn't get enough of studying them. Although their eye color was not as obvious as it is today, I could tell that Luke would have big, beautiful brown eyes. Whenever he looked at me, his gaze shot right through me, as if he were trying to talk to me. Layla's skin was almost impossibly delicate to the touch. Her soft smile and big bluish eyes lit up the twins' room. I still couldn't help but stroke their tiny fingers and tiny toes every chance I got.

A week later, Luke's breathing cannula was removed and he began breathing entirely on his own, although his feeding tube had to stay as he was still having difficulty drinking his bottle in the expected amount of time. Layla, on the other hand, was gulping down each feeding without any problem. She was still having severe episodes where she would not breathe, though. She needed more time with her cannula. The nurses would take it off, and she'd do well for a few hours, but then the tube would have to go right back on. One step forward, three steps back.

"This is expected," one nurse said. "As they rely more and more on their own lungs to breathe, they'll have more episodes for a while as they get used to not being on oxygen. It's like leveling up in a video game—when you get to the next level, you make a lot more mistakes."

Despite these fits and starts, hope continued to set in as the prospect of my babies coming home became more and more real. They continued to pass their routine scans, labs, head ultrasounds, and hearing tests. I even rescheduled my baby shower, which I had postponed once the twins were born prematurely, for April 28, confident that I could finally start arranging their nursery and preparing for their arrival. My life, which had stood still for what felt like countless months, was now starting to move in fast forward—that is, until I received a phone call from Luke's ophthalmologist.

april | jenny

CHAPTER 21

Seeing Eye to Eye

The evening of April 23, Joe and I were both at home. When the phone rang, I jumped in spite of myself.

"This is Luke's ophthalmologist," I heard on the other end of the line. "Luke's eye exam came back with stage three retinopathy of prematurity," she said.

"Stage three retinopathy—what does that mean?" I asked, feeling my heart beginning to pound.

"As you know, his weekly exams have consistently been stage one or stage two, which is usually no reason for concern. This week he has hit stage three. This means that the blood vessels are starting to grow into the center of the eye, which could cause loss of vision if they're left unattended. It's common in premature babies."

I froze. Just when I thought things were trending in the right direction...

143

"So, what are our options?" I asked.

"Time really is of the essence here. If we let his condition continue without intervention, there is a chance he could go blind. We are recommending immediate laser surgery to remove the blood vessels that could damage the retina."

Joe was in his office on the second floor of our house while I was having this conversation, but as soon as I heard the word "surgery," I said, "Let me go talk to my husband." I ran upstairs and filled him in on what the doctor had told me so far.

Both Joe and I wore glasses, but that couldn't compare to the fact that our son might lose his eyesight entirely. Although Luke and Layla had been having weekly eye exams every Tuesday to check for signs of this very issue, I obviously hadn't thought through the outside risks, even when the nurses had warned Joe and me not to visit during the exams. "It's a painful thing to watch," they explained. "It's not painful for the babies, but it *looks* painful. Most parents would rather not be there."

As I stood in Joe's office, I recalled a Tuesday morning when I had ignored the nurses' recommendations and ventured into the twins' room to see what these tests were all about.

The ophthalmologist gave them eye drops and then turned to leave the room. "I have to let the drops sit for 30 minutes to let them take effect," she explained. "They essentially numb their eyes and dilate their pupils so I can do my work."

When the doctor came back, I understood exactly why parents generally avoided this procedure. She pried open the twins' sealed eyelids with prongs and examined their retinae to look for any developing signs of abnormality in the blood vessels. Through Luke's and Layla's wide-open pupils, she snapped pictures of the backs of their eyes.

As the ophthalmologist finished the examination, she took off her gloves and turned to face me. "Layla's eyes are at stage one," she said, "That's normal. Luke's are at stage two right now, which is also normal, but we'll keep a close eye on him."

Even after all that, Joe and I still didn't know much about what stage three retinopathy looked like. We were so used to worrying about Luke's neurological development and immune system as a preemie that we hadn't considered the impact of his early birth on his eyesight.

"So, what do you think?" I heard the doctor say on the phone now, snapping me out of my reverie.

Although I couldn't imagine either of the twins having surgery at such a young age—their bodies were still so fragile and already enduring so much—Joe and I had no time to research the risks associated with it. We had no choice but to tell the ophthalmologist to move forward. If we didn't, and Luke lost his vision, how could we live with ourselves?

As tears began streaming down my face, Joe took the phone out of my hand. "Go ahead and do the laser treatment," he told the doctor.

As soon as he hung up, I wiped my eyes and said, "I'm going to the hospital right now. I have to be with Luke when he gets out."

By the time I arrived, Luke had already been taken out of the River room and sedated. When the procedure was over, he would stay in the Rainforest while he healed. I waited in an adjacent, cave-like room, with nothing in it besides the same green recliner, while his medical team worked on him. *Is this even going to work?* I wondered. *Is Luke going to have to see an ophthalmologist throughout his childhood? Will he need glasses? What if the laser burns his abnormal blood vessels and he loses his peripheral vision?* And, worst of all, *What if my son goes blind?* It didn't help when I Googled "retinopathy of prematurity" and discovered that Stevie Wonder, who was also a preemie and had lost his eyesight, had retinopathy of prematurity just like Luke had.

The procedure was relatively quick, and when a nurse came in to debrief me, she said, "Everything went well. Luke's doing fine. He's still sedated and not in any pain. He'll be in here shortly." But when they wheeled him into the Rainforest, back in an enclosed incubator, I couldn't help but fixate on how much he seemed to have regressed physically. He was hooked up to wires and an IV drip. He had a blue eye mask on, which is what he had worn as a newborn to block any light from reaching his eyes, and he was noticeably swollen. As soon as the doctors cleared me to hold him, I rocked him gently into the morning, whispering, "I would do anything to take your pain away, buddy. I will love you no matter what," I said, stroking his face. "Your father and I want the best for you, and we promise this is the best decision for you in the long run. We want you to be able to see the whole wide, wonderful world that's waiting for you out there."

I continued to rock him and hold him tight as he lay on my chest in a peaceful sleep. Finally, I had to head home to take Angelina to school. When I returned to the NICU, he was already back in the River room with Layla.

On April 28, although only five days had passed since Luke's surgery, I had my long-awaited baby shower. My mom and my best friend hosted 30 guests, all women, at my mom's house. We gathered in the living room, chatting and eating, and when the time came to open gifts, Angelina stayed close beside me, unwrapping each one and exclaiming over the adorable out-fits and toys my friends and relatives had bought me. Some of the guests were people I hadn't seen since Luke and Layla were born, but I didn't feel like I had to explain so much this time. I was optimistic that things were going well, and I was excited for my babies to come home, so the whole gathering felt authentically celebratory.

Once the shower was over, I also felt ready to continue decorating the twins' nursery, which still had only a chair and two cribs in it. Now, I put all the gifts I had received in the room. I stacked diapers and wipes on the changing table and placed the twins' new preemie clothes in the drawers and the closet. When I finished, I sat down in the rocker and smiled at the finished product. *Their room is ready for them to come home now. It will be soon. I can feel it.*

CHAPTER 22

Easter Blessings

When Jenny and I first heard that Luke needed laser surgery, we were in shock. I remember thinking, *You're seriously going to use lasers on a five-pound baby's eyes?* But the twins' ophthalmologist took the time to explain to us how common and relatively uncomplicated this procedure actually was, the advantages of doing it immediately versus the potential risks of waiting, and the high likelihood that Luke would be okay. After that, we believed we had the information we needed to validate our decision to move forward.

Sure enough, Luke seemed to bounce back quickly after his ordeal. And even without his oxygen cannula, he was still able to sustain breathing on his own throughout this touch-and-go situation.

"We are so blessed to have such dedicated doctors and nurses on our team," I said to the twins' doctor one day.

"Your professionalism and care for these fragile and vulnerable newborns is unbelievable. It takes a special personality—so much patience and resilience—to care for these babies. We can't thank you and your staff enough."

"Well, thank you. I'm flattered," the doctor said. He was always humble, but his smile told me how much my compliments pleased him.

He wasn't the only medical professional we had formed a bond with. Over our months at the hospital, we had become close to many of the staff, who all did their jobs with consummate finesse. Each NICU baby had their own nurse for every 12-hour shift, and the neonatologist would visit every few hours to check their vitals and make any necessary changes to their daily care regimen. They always carried special phones that would alert them when the babies' monitors went off so they could rush to their side.

Certain nurses built an extra-special connection with not only Luke and Layla but with Joe and me as well. They began to learn their personalities, the positions they preferred to sleep in, and their triggers.

"I can tell already, Luke is going to be such a handsome boy," one nurse said. "And Layla is going to be a feisty one. She's a real fighter for sure."

Every time Jenny and I heard genuinely caring remarks like these, we knew we were right to trust these people with our children's lives.

Easter was the first big holiday that we celebrated after the babies' birth. Jenny's faith, an ever-present part of her family and her upbringing, was stronger than ever during this time, and despite my earlier, tenuous relationship with God, my own faith had continued to grow tremendously. Jenny and I prayed every day for our children's health and well-being.

We typically spent Easter with our entire extended family, but this Easter was different. Jenny and I had to split our time between being with the twins in the morning and then spending the afternoon with her side of the family, along with my sister. She had recently had a baby of her own, a girl, in March, and was dealing with the sleeplessness and stress of having a newborn at home.

That Easter morning marked another milestone, as the twins were able to sit together on a play mat for the first time. Luke wore a blue-and-white-striped short-sleeved onesie, and Layla had on pink long-sleeved pajamas with cat faces on them. It was the closest they had been physically since they were in the womb, and the first time Jenny and I felt as if we were "back to normal." We propped them up on boppies covered in soft flannel hospital blankets for tummy time, watched as they smiled and wiggled their arms and legs around, and marveled at how much bigger and more alert they had become.

After we let them play and gave them a chance to just *be* babies, the way they always should have been, it was time to put them back in their cribs. It was hard to leave the hospital, especially on such a special day, but we knew they were in good hands and Angelina needed normalcy. She needed to be with her cousins, to feel joyful, and to burn off energy running around Vovó's house and her big backyard, as the kids loved to do. And any guilt that Jenny and I felt about leaving Luke and Layla was offset by being alongside family; lots of lamb, potatoes, and roast beef; painting Easter eggs; and hunting for them in the backyard.

My parents were not able to be with us because they were in Portugal. They lived in the same small city, only 15 minutes apart, but since their separation they had managed never to run into each other.

Regardless, where my parents remained aligned was in their love of their grandchildren. We FaceTimed with each of them daily, and their need for these regular updates was genuine. They had supported Jenny and Angelina and me from the first day of the twins' lives—giving us words of encouragement, praying for all of us, always wanting to know what was going on. Honestly, it was refreshing to see this positive side of my mom and dad, which I had always longed for.

CHAPTER 23

United at Once

———

By May, the sun was shining more, the days were longer, and spring was in the air. It had been a long flu season, but it was coming to a close, and the doctors had told us that once Luke and Layla's risk of influenza had subsided, Angelina would finally get to meet them in the hospital. I thought all the time about what her face would look like when she saw them for the first time, and I yearned for a family photo of all of us together—one that mimicked the drawings Angelina had been making in the hopes that our shared dream would come to life one day.

On May 13, I picked Angelina up from school. She hopped into her car seat, as she always did, with a big smile on her face.

"Guess what?" I said, as I buckled her in.

"What?"

"Your brother and sister are finally big enough and strong enough for you to see them. What do you say? Are you up for a visit?"

"Yes!" she shouted.

"I thought you would say that! Let's go. Dad is going to meet us there."

Joe and I had always told her this day would come, but I realize now that we weren't certain until the moment the doctor actually cleared her to come visit.

Angelina and I rushed over to the hospital and were greeted by Joe before we met with the nurses. They had told Joe and me ahead of time that they had a station for little kids where they would teach Angelina how to prepare for meeting her siblings. When we arrived, they were waiting for us in a meeting room just off the NICU—the very same meeting room where, the previous week, I had started making a scrapbook of our NICU journey. The nurses had laid everything out on the table—a stethoscope, a miniature blood pressure cuff, an oxygen cannula, a gown, and sterile gloves—and were ready to give Angelina a short demonstration of what she might see in the twins' hospital room. It was a lot for a five-year-old to comprehend, but a much-needed discussion.

I could tell Angelina was nervous because of her pinched smile. *She probably thinks this is some kind of setup*, I realized. But as soon as one of the nurses, a bubbly, joyous woman who looked like she lived for this kind of thing, said, "You must be Angelina. I hear you like art," that was all the icebreaker those two needed. Angelina's eyes lit up when the nurse asked, "How would you like to decorate these white preemie shirts for Luke and Layla any way you wish?" Seeing my daughter's eagerness, the nurse added, "Here are some stencils, markers, glitter, and other things you can use. I bet they'll love whatever you make them. Once you're finished with that, we can talk about all the fun stuff you see here on the table."

While Joe looked on and smiled, Angelina and I sat down in two small chairs and quickly got down to doing what she did best. She asked the nurse questions like "Can I use this color?" and "Can I paint this shirt?" We stenciled *NICU Warrior* on Luke's shirt and two beautiful butterflies on Layla's. She colored them in and left them to dry.

Next, Angelina listened closely while the nurse began to explain every detail about what she might see when she entered her brother and sister's room. "Do you know what this is? Do you know what it does and why we have it?" the nurse asked, holding up the blood pressure cuff. "Why do you think your brother and sister are in the NICU? Are you excited for them to come home?"

"Yes!" Angelina said.

"Great! Now, let's try the stethoscope on Mommy," the nurse said.

Angelina put it around her neck and in her ears. As I knelt to her level, she put the node on my heart and listened carefully.

"Now you're ready to be a doctor!" the nurse said. "When you walk into Luke and Layla's room, you'll understand some of the things you'll see."

"I can't wait!" Angelina said.

"Then let's get down there so you can meet your brother and sister."

The nurse beamed as she helped Angelina put on her yellow gown and white gloves. "This gown is to protect the babies," she explained. "We want to make sure we don't bring in any germs from the outside."

Angelina was so petite that her gown reached almost to the floor. I tied it up in the back so it wouldn't drag. We all practically floated down the hall. When we reached the River room, we let Angelina go in first; Joe followed close behind her, capturing every moment by taking a video on his phone.

Angelina looked at both ends of the room, one crib on each side. The large windows filled the room with sunlight. Joe steered her over to Luke's crib first, saying, "Mr. Luke's over here. Hi, Mr. Luke. Your big sister is here to meet you."

When Angelina peeked into Luke's crib, he looked right up at her with his big eyes.

"He's so cute!" she said. She watched as I gently picked him up and brought him closer to her. Angelina beamed as she and her brother stared at each other.

"Why don't you go meet your baby sister now?" I said after a minute, as I walked over to the green recliner to take a seat.

She raced to the other side of the room and met her sister. Layla was swaddled tightly, sleeping on her tummy, sucking on her pacifier. "Aw, she is adorable!" Angelina said.

"I'm so happy you can finally see them," I said, furtively wiping tears of joy from my eyes. *Finally, this is happening. Angelina is so happy right now. But what is she thinking and feeling right now? Is this too much for her? She's such a mature little girl; she seems thrilled to be meeting them.*

The nurses maneuvered Layla's wires to the center of the room as far as they could go before they stretched thin. The green recliners met in the middle. Joe reached for Layla, then sat down next to Luke and me.

Angelina perched on the edge of Joe's recliner and smiled for the first picture of us together as a family. We stayed in that moment for as long as we could, until it was time to put the twins back in their cribs.

Before we left the hospital, the nurse handed Angelina a pink shirt that read *Best Big Sister Ever*, along with a printed big sister award.

"Thank you!" she said.

She was happy. I was happy. Finally, in this moment, we were all so happy.

CHAPTER 24

Rebirth

Wind gusted across my face as my feet pounded the trail. The 30-pound backpack I was carrying felt like nothing. Recently, I had gotten into an activity called rucking, which involves walking at a brisk pace with a heavy weight on your back. I had already worked my way up from 10 pounds to 30 pounds and could tell I was growing stronger every day—not only physically, but also mentally and emotionally.

I liked to ruck around the lakes near our house, reflecting on my life and my family's situation, praying that my children would be healthy, listening to music, and often stopping to meditate. I read the book *Meditations* by Marcus Aurelius, and I started learning more about the law of attraction and the power of manifesting; that led me to explore books by motivational speakers such as Jordan Peterson and Ryan Holiday. Through my earbuds, I heard their voices encouraging me as I hurried along the path. Their words pushed me to keep going, to keep moving forward with the right mindset, and to recognize that by changing my attitude, I would change my altitude.

This was me—the new me. I had always fought for others. That had never been difficult for me. But now I had to fight for myself, in order to be the best father possible to Angelina and to Luke and Layla. It all started when I got down on my knees in the hospital right before they were born and prayed that they would survive. I said to myself, *Either I am going to break down or I am going to find every possible way to turn an exhausting and traumatic situation into a pivotal moment that changes who I am at a core level and gives me the motivation to go out and have a healthy heart, mind, and soul.*

I started giving myself the same pieces of wise advice I had always offered freely to my friends and family. And when I still felt stressed, I went to the gym, lifted weights, and did cardio. If I didn't have time to work out, I spent some time with the punching bag in my garage, letting out my anxiety, or I meditated to try to relax.

That didn't mean it was a perfect evolution. I frequently had to summon the courage to keep going when my anxiety started playing with my head and doubt took over: *You won't be able to be a good dad to them. You'll never finish school. Your marriage will fall apart.* I had to somehow remove this nonsense and think positively. *Look at all that I've accomplished. I went back to school. I started my own business. I'm managing all that while my babies fight day in and day out in the hospital. Why am I doubting myself?*

I wasn't always able to dismiss these thorny thoughts, but I was learning to adapt. To be patient. Everything is a process— like the twins' healing. My children taught me that, along with patience. It takes time for things to evolve and bloom the way they're supposed to. And after all that Jenny and I have been through, I have proven to myself that I am tough. My wife is one of the strongest people I know, and our three kids are the toughest of us all. Jenny had taken these last few months completely in stride, keeping her head up and keeping us all on the right path of staying positive. I could tell she was bottling up a lot of her emotions inside but always had the strength to prevent anything from knocking her down.

In fact, all parents are tougher than many of us ever realize, and all humans have it in us to survive. Life throws a curveball and smacks us in the face with situations we think we can't handle—until we have no choice but to handle them. We can either give up, falling toward our weak side, or hunker down and push forward. And that is the greatest gift we can give to our children: our own courageous selves, which live and lead by example.

In late April, Layla mastered bottle feeding and got her feeding tube removed. A few weeks later, close to the twins' original due date of May 5, her oxygen cannula was removed. We were so close. In order for Layla to come home, she just had to breathe consistently on her own, without setting off any alarms, for five days straight.

One evening shortly after that, I arrived at the hospital and one of the new doctors said, "Good news! Layla will be ready to go home soon! She's gone a few days without an episode, and she seems to be doing well breathing on her own. As long as everything goes okay tonight, we'll release her tomorrow morning."

I wanted to respond with a big smile, a cheer, a sigh of relief, but I couldn't do that yet because, ever since Layla's team had removed her nasal cannula, Jenny and I had been concerned. She was still frequently having breathing episodes, even in her sleep. A few doctors had said this was a normal part of adjusting to life without the machines, but all Jenny and I could remember were the fear and the panic we had experienced each time Layla had to be resuscitated, which was more than once. As much as we wanted our babies to come home with us, we would have been terrified if something had happened on our watch, and we couldn't even imagine the fallout if Angelina had to witness such a scare. So, even if Layla's medical team was comfortable sending her home, we weren't ready, and we didn't think Layla was ready either.

So, as soon as the doctor walked out, I called Jenny and said, "Her original neonatologist told me a few weeks ago that she had to be free and clear of alarms for five straight days, and that seven days would be even better, but right now I don't think it's time yet."

"She's not going home tomorrow," Jenny agreed. "She's been having some acid reflux lately, which has been causing her to relapse, and all her spitting up is causing her to lose weight. She still has a lot of episodes, way more than Luke. Sometimes I even wish they would put the cannula back in."

After I hung up with Jenny, I walked over to Layla's crib, my chest tight. I was almost ready to cry. She lay peacefully, wrapped tightly in her blanket. I reached into the crib and grabbed her hand.

"Layla, if you're not ready to go home, you need to tell us. Tonight's the night. Give us a sign." I also offered up a silent prayer in the room: *Don't let her come home if she's not ready. If she has an episode and sounds the alarm, the hospital will have to keep her here for five more days.*

That evening, after putting everything in the hands of someone more powerful than I was, I was shocked at how peaceful I felt. "You've taught me so much," I whispered into the dark. "I wasn't like this before you two were born. I thought I could fix everything. But now I know I can't, and that's okay. I can trust—and rest."

At three o'clock that morning, Layla had an episode— then another, then another. When Jenny updated me the next morning, she said, "She's not going home today. The hospital reported three episodes in one night. They officially can't release her for another five days."

"That's what I thought," I said, exhaling a silent prayer of relief and gratitude. *Thank you, Layla. I knew you could do it.*

Over the next few weeks, our original doctor, who had been with the twins since admission, reassured us, "They can stay as long as they need to, until we all agree it's safe for them to go home. We changed her formula to help with the weight gain and the acid reflux. Those refluxes were causing the episodes. We are optimistic that she'll feel better soon."

I nodded. "One more thing," I said. "When Layla does go home, Jenny asked if you can send a monitor with us so that we can actually sleep at night. It's going to be terrifying for us if she decides not to breathe."

"Absolutely," the doctor said. "We'll give you an apnea monitor for Layla to wear 24/7 for a couple weeks, to give you peace of mind. You will tape down the leads on her chest, just like we do here in the NICU, and an alarm will sound and catch any sudden episodes if she stops breathing or if her heart rate drops for any reason. I also recommend that you, Jenny, and any other caregivers you plan to have around your babies take a CPR class so you're as prepared as you can be just in case the worst does occur."

"Thank you, Doctor," I said. "I'm not sure what we would have done without you."

CHAPTER 25

Home at Last

On May 20, after 115 long days in the NICU—and, coincidentally, on Joe's birthday—Layla was finally ready to come home. She had shown all of us that she could breathe on her own without help from nurses, doctors, or any level of manufactured oxygen. The apnea monitor Joe had requested from the twins' doctor would be only a precaution for the first few weeks.

Joe, my mom, and I had also all taken the CPR class our doctor had recommended. The March of Dimes helped coordinate the class at the hospital to assist parents in feeling more secure about bringing home NICU babies. We were as prepared as we could possibly be—but would that be enough?

That morning, Joe and I went to the hospital together and gathered all of Layla's belongings from her stay. We packed her very first hat, a blood pressure cuff that fit around my finger, a pacifier, and a few of her earliest diapers to remember how miniature she had been and how far she and her brother had come. I would add everything to their scrapbook—including the photo we took of Luke, Layla, Joe, and me when we were ready to take Layla home .

Layla passed her head ultrasound, hearing test, eye exam, and car seat challenge, in which she had to be a certain height and weight and be strapped in for 90 minutes without having a breathing episode. She was finally the size of a full-term baby. After that, we locked all six pounds of her tightly in her car seat, which engulfed her entire body. The leads extending from her apnea monitor were attached to her chest, tracking her every breath.

We had been living in this world day in and day out for the past 115 days. We had assumed that when we left it behind, we would have both babies with us. But Luke just wasn't quite ready to come home yet. On his side of the room, he lay swaddled, sleeping peacefully. He was breathing well, and by then he had made a full recovery from his eye surgery, but he still needed a feeding tube to ensure he was getting all the milk he wasn't able to get from the bottle. We had tried switching formulas, but none of them sat well in his stomach, and he was frequently spitting up and losing weight.

I gave Luke a big kiss before heading out with his sister. "We'll be back soon, buddy," I said. We needed to get home as quickly as possible so I could take Layla with me to pick up Angelina from school.

We walked out of the hospital room, Joe carrying Layla in her car seat, but I knew it wasn't for the last time. *This isn't exactly what I was picturing,* I thought, *but at least one of our babies is finally ready to leave this place, and I know her brother is right behind her. Any day now. And in the meantime, he's in good hands.*

When I got to school, I sat in the carpool line, waiting for Angelina. It was like any other day over the past several months, except today she was in for a real surprise. A squeaky, mewing sound came from the backseat as Layla wriggled in her car seat.

I turned around and smiled at her. "Your sister is going to be so surprised, isn't she, Layla?"

I spotted Angelina walking single-file out of the school door, behind her other classmates. Her teacher saw my car, nodded at her, and gave her a gentle nudge to dismiss her.

She walked toward the car, and her teacher opened the door to help her in. Then I heard her scream of delight.

"Layla! I'm so happy to see you!" she said as she climbed into the backseat and buckled herself into the car seat next to her sister. Then she paused, looking around. "Where's Luke?"

Nothing gets past this kid, I thought.

"He's still at the hospital," I said. "He's not quite ready to come home yet, but soon. In the meantime, let's get you girls home so we can get Layla settled in her new room and celebrate Daddy's birthday with some cake!"

When we pulled up in front of the house, I carefully unbuckled Layla's car seat, gathered up her apnea monitor and its attached wires, and followed Angelina as she practically danced into the house. All afternoon, Angelina didn't leave Layla's side. Whenever I needed something—a diaper, a wipe, a rag to clean up projectile vomit—Angelina jumped up to get it. "I'll bring you whatever you need," she would say with a smile, and I knew she was doing it because she wanted to, not because she had to. After all, this was what she had always wanted.

My parents had met us at home to be there for Layla's arrival.

My mom, who had been present for every step of the journey, was especially emotional on this day. "My grandchildren make my life full of love. When you're old, they become your life; you need them to keep you going. They bring us so much joy. I'm just so happy Layla is finally home," she said, her eyes full of tears. "Now we just need Luke here with us. But I'll never forget the time I spent with them in the hospital."

"I'll never forget it either, Mom," I said, clasping her hand.

My father, who has a hard outer shell but is a teddy bear on the inside, melted when he saw Layla.

In his own way, he was consistently involved in Luke and Layla's early life. He called Joe and me out of the blue multiple times per week to check in on us and the babies. He was also close friends with a father of twins born prematurely 15 years earlier, so he was constantly calling him and inquiring about what to expect with Luke and Layla. And now that he was seeing Layla at my house, his delight was palpable. He was always so cautious at holding any of his 10 grandchildren as infants, and this time was no different, but he smiled at Layla and told me how beautiful she looked and how pretty her eyes were.

Joe's parents also each FaceTimed with us that day so that they could see Layla in her own home and wish their son a happy birthday. Their smiles practically burst through the screen. Joe's mother promised us she would visit as soon as she could make the trip overseas.

Still, it wasn't over. One piece of my heart was missing: Luke. On May 23, three days after Layla came home, the doctors were finally able to remove his feeding tube. We had found a formula that he could keep down, and he had grown into a strong, eight-pound, eight-ounce bundle of super-cuteness. The only remaining hurdle was that he was still having difficulty breathing and swallowing at the same time.

I had gone back to work while both babies were still in the hospital, but now that Layla had been discharged, my official full-time leave from work began. I struggled to divide my time between my infant at home and my infant at the hospital. Now that Layla was home, Joe and I didn't sleep and were on constant alert—and that was with only one infant. My mom stepped up even more and spent many hours helping out at our house. Joe went to see Luke at the NICU more frequently while I stayed home with Layla—he loved that father–son time, the long nights in the green recliner, bottle-feeding and rocking our boy to sleep—and I went whenever I had a chance.

There were some bright spots during that hectic time, mostly in the form of other visitors at the hospital; my brother and my sister-in-law came to see us, as did Joe's mother and a select few of our closest friends. But by the time they met Layla and Luke, they were the size of typical newborns, so our guests couldn't fathom what they had looked like at the beginning. It was also hard for people to get their heads around the idea that these babies were "five months adjusted" in age—significantly under the standard weight for full-term five-month-olds. To the world they looked and acted like newborns, when in reality, they were already 5 months old. We just had to focus on moving forward and on the love we would give our children for the rest of their lives.

Luke improved every day, and we soon began to feel as if we were going to the hospital only to feed him and watch him sleep. He had already passed his car seat challenge, and all his final exams came back free and clear.

"I think he's ready, Doc," I finally said. "Even if the current formula we're giving him doesn't end up working, I'd rather have him home with us, where he belongs."

"Okay," the doctor said. "As long as you feel comfortable feeding him at home, I'm willing to schedule his discharge."

On June 5, sixteen days after Layla came home and a month after the twins' due date, Luke was released. As with Layla's departure, we packed up his belongings, put him in his car seat, and said our goodbyes to the NICU staff. One of

Luke's nurses, the nurse who had received him on day one, was the same one who officially discharged him. I took a picture of her holding him while she told me how handsome he was and how much she was going to miss him.

As we carried Luke down the hall, we knew we weren't coming back—at least, we hoped not—but that realization was a bittersweet one, and a shock in itself. *This is it. We can't come back, because they're not going to let us, and even though this is what we wanted, it also means that our lives in the NICU for the past 130 days are over.* I realized, that in an odd way, we were going to miss this place, or maybe it was just the people inside it. The ones who cared not only for our babies but for all the other babies in the NICU. The ones who worked the night shift and stayed awake until morning in case a baby needed tending to. The ones who saved Luke's and Layla's lives.

We glanced one last time at the photos of NICU survivors that lined the corridor. I remembered our first day in this wing, I remembered the cries of the mother who had lost her baby here, and I had to steady myself in a moment of gratitude for how far we had come and for how fortunate we were, when others were not.

However, I also knew that even when both babies were home, Joe and I couldn't let our guard down. Layla had come home with the heart monitor we had requested in case she stopped breathing in the middle of the night. Luke still wasn't out of the woods; he still wasn't eating enough, and he had barely reached the weight desired for discharge. Joe and I would probably have PTSD from the hospital for a long time. But we believed that it was worth trying to have Luke with our family, in a new environment. As hard as all of this was going to be, it was time. Time to move on and raise these twins at home, alongside their sister. And I was up for the challenge. *If I survived the past five months, I sure as hell can survive what's in front of me*, I reminded myself.

We drove Luke home and placed him in Layla's crib, right next to her. I had to see the two of them finally together, in our own house, with nothing holding them apart—a sight that had seemed inconceivable five months earlier.

Angelina soon got home from school with my mom and ran upstairs to the nursery.

"Luke!" she squealed. "You're home, too! Mom, I'm so happy they're both finally here!"

I smiled. My cute, intuitive, talkative little girl. "Me too, sweetie."

That first evening, I sat in the nursery with Angelina, looking up at a sign I had hung. It read *Sometimes Miracles Come in Pairs*. Our house was complete. Layla was lying in her crib, the one that had stood empty for so long, the one I had gazed at longingly countless times over the past few months. Luke was in my arms, drinking his milk.

My mind wandered to the moments right before we had left the hospital. We were all home, but we were not entirely out of the woods. The babies' NICU doctor had briefed us on what to expect after taking them home. The twins would need multiple follow-ups with various specialists. Nurses would visit our home, and Luke and Layla would need regular occupational therapy, physical therapy, pulmonology checkups, and eye and hearing exams for the first six months to a year. Even though flu season had passed, the doctor gave us strict instructions about keeping them away from germs and limiting the number of visitors who came into the house.

"Luke and Layla did remarkably well for having been born 14 weeks early, and they both fought every day until the end of their NICU stay. These are the happy endings we NICU doctors and nurses work so hard for and why we love what we do. Your triumphant story makes it all worth it," said their neonatologist.

He continued, "For the first two years of their life, their lungs and immune systems will be fragile. It's important to keep them away from large crowds and smoke. Use very good hand hygiene, and always be conscious and careful with them. The last thing you want is to end up right back at this hospital. We're always happy to see you—but for a visit. We don't want to see you guys as patients here ever again!" he finished with a wink. I couldn't have agreed more.

"We'll do our best to keep them safe," I assured him.

"I know you will," he said. "Now comes the hard part: raising them, which unfortunately isn't something we can help you with." He laughed.

When Joe came home from work and joined the four of us in the nursery, Luke and Layla were both sleeping peacefully in their cribs. As he, Angelina, and I stared at them, I knew Joe was thinking something similar to the realization I had had earlier in the hospital: *I cannot believe we made it through this. That they made it through this. They are so beautiful, and I am so grateful they are both healthy. They're home. Now let's get ready for the next leg of our journey, the next part of our story.* I also remembered my wish when I'd said goodbye to Angelina in the middle of the night, right before Joe and I had rushed to the hospital the previous January: *They look just as sweet and safe as their big sister did that night.*

I put my arms around my husband and my eldest daughter and granted myself one more moment of thanks: *This is everything I've been hoping and wishing for, for so long.* Through it all, we never gave up on our babies' survival and they never gave up on their fight for life. I never could have imagined that Joe and I would have to face an experience like this, but ultimately it was a gift and a true blessing, one that forced us to work together and made us stronger than we had ever been. We were and forever will be a family with an unbreakable bond.

Forever Changed

My life had become a revolving door within my new normal. After a five-month-long battle and roller coaster in the NICU, we now had to face the new challenges of having Luke and Layla at home and raising three kids. Of course, we were grateful for finally having them home, although on top of all the extra precautions we had to take, we came face-to-face with the realization: *Shit—we have twins at home now,* and *a five-year-old!* Even families that brought home full-term twins with no health issues and no other siblings could barely keep their heads above water. *After what we just went though, do we still have enough willpower in us to get through this next chapter in our lives?* we wondered.

Joe and I both had plenty of nightmares, not to mention false alarms when Layla's monitor woke us up in the middle of the night, before her pulmonologist told us that the leads were hooked up incorrectly, probably because of our fatigue. The twins were used to being woken up for feeding and care every three hours in the NICU—a ritual that was hard to break in order for us to get the sleep we needed so badly. There were periods when we didn't shower for a couple of days. We had no time to exercise or eat well. We were on constant alert, existing in a state of pure exhaustion. In a time when we needed all hands-on deck, the doctors insisted that we quarantine to keep the twins safe, shielding them from the outside world and allowing very few members of our inner circle to visit, because of the babies' vulnerability and our fear of germs or catching a respiratory infection like the flu or RSV.

We also had the endless series of follow-up visits with the specialists our doctor had referred us to in order to track the twins' development. There were routine visits with the ophthalmologist, pulmonologists, pediatrician and occupational therapists who came regularly to our house to track their developmental milestones: Were they able to roll over? Could they sit up on their own? Did they crawl when they were supposed to? My babies who were born at 26 weeks' gestation were now five-month-old babies but looked and moved like newborns. Thankfully, once the twins got home, they were always on track and didn't miss a beat; they just did what they needed to do, as if being preemies was a thing of the past. They continued to eat well and grew every day. They began crawling and doing all the things full-term babies should have been doing at their adjusted age. They were progressing so well that I got to the point where I told the therapist, "Thank you, but I really don't think your services are necessary anymore. I think they're doing fine," and she agreed.

After nine months of doctor appointments, quarantine, and no sleep, we were eager for the day when we could take Luke and Layla out of the house more and visit our loved ones. But in March 2020, the COVID-19 pandemic restarted the clock for us. We had already been housebound for so long, and had used so many gallons of hand sanitizer and worn so many disposable masks, that the CDC's recommendations for COVID protocols were nothing new for us, yet this became a new scare for all of us. The risk that any of our children could end up in the hospital continued to keep us up at night. The NICU had saved their lives, but it was now a place we strove to avoid.

Angelina continued to be the best big sister, lending a helping hand whenever Mom and Dad needed her. Thankfully, she slept through our walks back and forth down the hall, past her bedroom door, for nighttime feedings or babies crying, but she did have to be around during the constant daytime bottle feedings, spit-ups, and diaper changes.

Through all the sleepless nights and challenges that come with being parents, we never forget how thankful and how blessed we are to be where we are today. I can tell you from my own experience that a journey in the NICU will change you forever. It will hold a piece of your heart that is irreplaceable. It's a battle of ups, downs, stress, anxiety, and depression, but it can also be filled with tears of joy and hope. At first, you become emotionally numb, and then it becomes a string of emotions that sits with you the entire time your child is in there. You live in a permanent state of not knowing, unaware what the next day, hour, or even minute might bring.

The best-case scenario for a premature baby is to stay healthy in order to grow, fully develop, and learn to breathe and eat on their own. You can only hope that any complications that arise during a NICU stay are not grave or, worse, fatal. Fortunately, despite a few setbacks, I encountered the best-case scenario when the odds were not in my favor. Getting to the end of that road could have destroyed my family and me had circumstances been different. If you find yourself in a situation like mine, you will cry—a lot. You will be angry, upset, and confused, and you will find yourself sitting alone during a lot of dark days. Ask for guidance, and accept all the help you can get from your family, friends, and support groups—and if you don't have any, ask your hospital's staff to refer you to someone to talk with.

You must stay hopeful, find the strength that lives inside all of us, and have faith that you will eventually start shedding tears of joy rather than pain and experience true happiness.

They say God never gives us more than we can handle, and that we have to stay calm, try to be patient, and take things one step at a time. And, eventually, we realize that priceless gifts can emerge from this state of deep uncertainty. I learned a lot during this experience, which was a reminder of the true meaning of family. I learned what and who is important in life. I don't sweat the small stuff anymore; now, I focus on what matters. The forever scar on my belly that once frightened me so much is now a representation of my struggle to find strength I never knew I had, and will always be a symbol of the miracles in my life and of my family's triumphant story.

I remember days when I truly believed I was not going to make it through. But I did. We all did, through a lot of hope, faith, and perseverance.

Acknowledgments

Writing this story was not easy and quite the journey, one that has helped me cope with the trauma that I experienced during such a challenging time. I never gave up on finishing this book, because I wanted to leave a legacy for my children, and I truly hope and believe that one day our powerful story might help shed a light on someone else's dark days.

To my book editors and designers, thank you for your creativity and for understanding my story, seeing my vision and making this book come alive.

I express great gratitude to the entire Women's Center and NICU hospital staff. You were an incredible team that provided expert care and nurturing support for my entire family. I will be forever indebted to the nurses, surgeons, and neonatologists who saved not only my life but the lives of my babies.

Your dedication to our health and safety was exceptional and unforgettable. In addition, I want to acknowledge the March of Dimes organization, who advocate and dedicate their time to supporting families with infants in the NICU. Your presence and the resources, education, and activities that you provided were and still are invaluable to me. I applaud you for the work you do for your mission.

Thank you to my in-laws, and all our family members and friends who were our support group, our shoulders to cry on, and who continuously offered prayers and words of encouragement. The many gestures did not go unnoticed and will never be forgotten. I hope you know who you are.

A special thank you to my mom and dad. Without your daily support, I would have fallen to pieces. Growing up, you both taught me that life is not always perfect, but that you must be strong, have faith and keep moving. Mom, you stood by my side, saw things that no grandmother should see her grandkids go through, and never gave up hope. Your prayers and countless hours by my side at the hospital went a long way. Your guidance and nurturing demeaner is what I strive to mimic for my children, and I am truly blessed to call you mom.

To my husband, Joe: We made it. Now we have an unbreakable bond that only you and I will truly understand. Thank you for helping me tell our story. Thank you for being my pillar and for your strength to push through such difficult times. I am grateful that the magnitude of our stress did not let us lose focus of what was important. Our story does not end here.

To Angelina, my firstborn, my beautiful soul. The strength and grace you showed at just five years old during such a difficult time was an unbelievable sight. Your unwavering spirit and gentle heart made the toughest times easier, and for that, I am eternally grateful. You truly are amazing—never forget that. I pray that your light continues to shine bright.

Luke and Layla, my precious miracle babies. You both are an inspiration and you are living proof to the world that anything is possible. Your birth as a premature baby does not define who you are but shows that you came into this world fighting and highlights the incredible strength and determination within you. I hope your will to persevere will carry on throughout your lives, knowing that you are destined to leave a mark on this world.

To all three of my children. Thank you for reminding me every day of how incredibly blessed I am. Life is fragile, and I thank God every day for the privilege of being your mother. Know that your dad and I love you more than words can express, and it is our duty to guide you to become the best versions of yourselves. We hope that one day when you read this story you will learn that in moments of defeat or when faced with challenges, you must never give up and always believe in yourself to persevere.

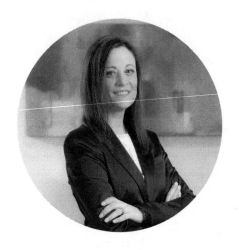

Meet the Author

Jennifer is a first-generation Portuguese American who authored her first book, *Week 26* aspiring to help others, all while leaving a legacy for her children. She received her bachelor's degree from George Mason University and was once a journalist on a kids' television show. When she's not working or spending time with her family and friends, she's surrounded by her pets, listening to music or enjoying the outdoors. Her life is fueled by her children, her family, and her culture, all of which have made her who she is today.

www.week26.com

Made in the USA
Columbia, SC
09 October 2024

64cdf880-0cac-4e95-94dc-a79c54da8789R01